T0176741

A Practical Approach to Using Statistics in Health Research

A Practical Approach to Using Statistics in Health Research

From Planning to Reporting

Adam Mackridge
Philip Rowe

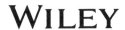

Registered Office
John Wiley & Sons, Inc., 111 River Street, Hoboken, NJ 07030, USA

Editorial Office
111 River Street, Hoboken, NJ 07030, USA

For details of our global editorial offices, customer services, and more information about Wiley products visit us at www.wiley.com.

Wiley also publishes its books in a variety of electronic formats and by print-on-demand. Some content that appears in standard print versions of this book may not be available in other formats.

Library of Congress Cataloguing-in-Publication Data
Names: Mackridge, Adam (Adam John), 1979- author. | Rowe, Philip, author.
Title: A practical guide to statistics for health research / by Adam
    Mackridge, Philip Rowe.
Description: Hoboken, NJ : Wiley, 2018. | Includes bibliographical references
    and index. |
Identifiers: LCCN 2017055955 (print) | LCCN 2018001635 (ebook) | ISBN
    9781119383598 (pdf) | ISBN 9781119383611 (epub) | ISBN 9781119383574
    (hardback)
Subjects: LCSH: Medical statistics. | Medicine–Research–Statistical
    methods. | BISAC: MEDICAL / Epidemiology. | MATHEMATICS / Probability &
    Statistics / General.
Classification: LCC R853.S7 (ebook) | LCC R853.S7 M33 2018 (print) | DDC
    610.2/1–dc23
LC record available at https://lccn.loc.gov/2017055955

Cover Design: Wiley
Cover Image: © Tetra Images/Getty Images

Set in 10/12pt WarnockPro by SPi Global, Chennai, India

Printed in the United States of America

10 9 8 7 6 5 4 3 2 1

Contents

About the Companion Website

This book is accompanied by Student companion websites:

www.wiley.com/go/Mackridge/APracticalApproachtoUsing StatisticsinHealthResearch

The website is aimed at helping readers of our book to understand how to use statistical tests correctly in their research. It is aimed at people working in health or social care who are interested in carrying out research and recognise the importance of statistical testing to provide robustness to the analysis and credibility to the findings. The book describes how to tackle the statistics for most common scenarios where the study design is fairly simple. The book is intended to help you **use** statistics in practice-focussed research and will not attempt to provide a full theoretical background to statistical methods. For that, you can turn to our sister publication (Rowe, 2015).

The book, supported by the materials on the website, set out the basic rules for using statistical tests, guides the reader through the process of deciding which test is most appropriate to their project and then provides a stepwise description of how to use the test.

The website contains three main components:

1. A checklist to help you determine which is the most appropriate test you're your project
2. Videos showing how to use key software (G*Power and SPSS) to determine sample sizes and carry out statistical analysis
3. The data files that we have taken examples from, so that you can see the raw data and try to replicate the tests that we have applied – if you get the same results as us, it's an excellent indication that you've got the hang of using the test

We have also provided SPSS data files where this software has been used in our examples. If you do not have access to this software, the instructions should still be useful; all packages work in essentially similar ways. The choice of statistical routine, the information you have to supply to allow the method to run correctly and the key pieces of output that you have to identify will not vary from package to package.

To allow you to do this, we have also provided the data in MS Excel format so that you can access this and copy it into the statistical programme of your choice. If you do not have access to MS Excel, you can open the files in MS Excel Viewer (available from www.microsoft.com).

1

Introduction

1.1   At Whom is This Book Aimed?

There are countless people working in areas related to health who are, or could be, involved in research. This certainly includes doctors, dentists, nurses, pharmacists, physiotherapists, midwives, and health visitors, but there are many other groups where this is equally true. The types of useful research they could be carrying out range from simple descriptions of the frequency of a particular condition in a specific location or describing local adherence to a health guideline through to more complex work involving comparisons between groups of patients, organizations, or geographical locales, etc. Based on our experience, one hurdle to involvement in carrying out this type of research is a lack of confidence in using statistics. This book is aimed at that group of health workers who are interested in building the evidence base to underpin excellent practice in their area, but who are struggling to design good quality analyses that stand up to scrutiny. It focuses on what you need to know to use statistics correctly to improve the robustness of your project without all of the theory and complex mathematics. It is not intended for anybody who already has significant research experience or for those who aim to become expert statisticians.

Our assumption is that any project our would-be researcher undertakes will be fairly simple. We use the word "simple" advisedly. We do not use it to imply triviality or that such work is necessarily easy. By "simple," we mean the opposite of complex. It can be very tempting to investigate simultaneously six different factors that

A Practical Approach to Using Statistics in Health Research: From Planning to Reporting, First Edition. Adam Mackridge and Philip Rowe.
© 2018 John Wiley & Sons, Inc. Published 2018 by John Wiley & Sons, Inc.
Companion website: www.wiley.com/go/Mackridge/
APracticalApproachtoUsingStatisticsinHealthResearch

might influence a particular clinical outcome or indeed to look at numerous outcomes for a given factor. Such complexity all too often leads to a tangled mass of data that defies clear interpretation. In order to produce clear and robust evidence, it is important to keep it simple and look at questions such as, whether people living in the more deprived part of your local town suffer increased levels of a particular condition, or whether patients counseled by nurses have a better understanding of their medication than those counseled by doctors. By keeping your design simple, as in these latter cases, any positive finding will be easily and unambiguously interpretable and much more likely to help develop best practice. Our motto is "Keep it simple – keep it clear." In line with this philosophy, the statistical methods covered in this book are deliberately limited to those that consider the possibility that a single factor might have some influence upon a single clinical outcome.

1.2   At What Scale of Project is This Book Aimed?

The type of research project for which we envisage this book being useful is quite small: typically involving one or two researchers or something handled by a small team, with you, the reader, as the leader or a prominent member of the project team. Large, complex studies that involve significant funding (e.g. those funded by the UK's National Institute for Health Research) would almost certainly require the services of a specialist statistician, at which point this book becomes more of a guide to help you understand the techniques that may be used and the reasons for this, but it would be unlikely to cover all the statistical aspects of your project.

1.3   Why Might This Book be Useful for You?

The intention is to provide a handbook – something you can pick up, read the bit you need, and put down. You do not need to read it from cover to cover. It provides "how to" advice that covers the complete journey through a research project. How to:

- Work out how much data you need to collect in order to provide a reliable answer to the question you have asked (sample size).

- Identify an appropriate measure of effect size, and use that to determine whether any difference you have detected is large enough to be of practical significance (i.e. is a change in public policy or professional practice required?)
- Identify appropriate statistical methods.
- Apply the relevant statistical methods to your data using statistical software, mainly using SPSS.
- Identify which bits of the software output you need to focus on and how to interpret them.
- Determine whether your data indicates statistical significance (i.e. is there adequate evidence that outcomes really do differ between the groups studied?)
- Determine whether your data indicates practical/clinical significance (i.e. is any difference between study groups big enough to be of practical consequence?)
- Make sure any publications you write contain all the necessary statistical details.

This book is intended to help you **use** statistics in practice-focused research and will not attempt to provide a full theoretical background to statistical methods. For that, you can turn to our sister publication (Rowe, 2015).[1]

1.4 How to Use This Book

Table 1.1 shows the ideal flow of events from first planning stages through to final analysis and reporting of your experimental data. It may not always be possible to adhere to every detail, but this describes an ideal approach, at which to aim.

Everybody should read the first six chapters of this book.
You can than select the appropriate chapter from the remainder of the book, which will talk you through sample size planning, execution of the statistical test, and interpretation and reporting of the results.

Chapter 20 describes Cronbach's alpha. This is not a statistical test as such but is covered in a short chapter due to its widespread use in questionnaire-based research.

---

[1] Rowe P. Essential statistics for the pharmaceutical sciences, 2nd edn. Chichester: Wiley, 2015.

Table 1.1 The ideal stage-by-stage flow of events for a research program.

Stage	Actions	Chapters to read
1	Identify the research question that is to be answered.	
2	Make an outline plan of an experiment/trial/ survey that will answer the question.	
3	Decide which statistical test you will use.	2, 3, and 4
4	Determine the smallest effect size you want to be able to detect.	
5	Using the results from steps three and four, calculate appropriate sample sizes.	Relevant chapter from 7 to 20
6	Perform the survey/experiment etc.	
7	Describe the data obtained.	Chapter 3 and relevant
8	Carry out the test selected at step three, and draw your conclusions as to statistical and practical/ clinical significance.	chapter from 7 to 20
9	If other interesting features emerged within the results, analyze these, but report them as exploratory (or secondary) analyses and do not place undue reliance on any conclusions.	Relevant chapter from 7 to 20
10	Consider whether you have increased the risk of generating false positive findings by carrying out multiple statistical tests.	5
11	Report your findings.	Relevant chapter from 7 to 20

1.5 Computer Based Statistics Packages

This book and its accompanying videos concentrate mainly on SPSS, as this is probably the most widely used package in health research. If you do not have access to SPSS, the instructions should still be useful; all packages work in essentially similar ways. The choice of statistical routine, the information you have to supply to allow the method to run correctly, and the key pieces of output that you have to identify will not vary from package to package.

On our companion website, we have provided all of our data files in SPSS format, but in case you do not have access to this, we have also provided the data in Microsoft Excel format. If you do not have access to this program either, you can download a free Excel Viewer program from Microsoft's website that will allow you to view the data sets.

Unfortunately, despite its considerable price, SPSS does not calculate necessary sample sizes. We therefore also refer to G*Power, which will do this job. G*Power is free software that can be downloaded from the internet – we would advise using the Heinrich-Heine-Universität Düsseldorf site.

1.6   Relevant Videos etc.

The practical execution of statistical routines using SPSS is covered in a collection of videos. Individual chapters indicate where you can view these.

The following video, relevant to this chapter, is available at www.wiley.com/go/Mackridge/APracticalApproachtoUsingStatisticsin HealthResearch

Video_1.1_SPSS_Basics: The absolute basics of using SPSS.

2

Data Types

2.1 What Types of Data are There and Why Does it Matter?

Before you can select a statistical method, you will need to identify what types of data you plan to collect. The choice of descriptive and analytical methods depends crucially on the type of data involved. There are three types:

- Continuous measured/Scale (such as blood pressure measured in mmHg).
- Ordinal (such as a Likert scale – Strongly disagree to Strongly agree).
- Categorical/Nominal (such as which ward a patient is on).

The first two types are concerned with the *measurement* of some characteristic. The final type is just a classification with no sense of measurement.

2.2 Continuous Measured Data

This is also known as "Interval" or "Scale" data. Clinical observations often produce continuous measured data: these include weights, volumes, timings, concentrations, pressures, etc. The important aspects of this type of data are:

- The characteristic being assessed varies continuously. For example, we measure blood pressure using discrete steps of one mmHg, but

A Practical Approach to Using Statistics in Health Research: From Planning to Reporting, First Edition. Adam Mackridge and Philip Rowe.
© 2018 John Wiley & Sons, Inc. Published 2018 by John Wiley & Sons, Inc.
Companion website: www.wiley.com/go/Mackridge/
APracticalApproachtoUsingStatisticsinHealthResearch

the reality is that pressure could be 91.25 mmHg (or any figure with an unlimited number of decimal places) – we just choose not to measure to this degree of precision.

- There is a large number of possible different values that might be recorded. For example, diastolic blood pressures typically vary over a range of 60 to 120 mmHg, giving 61 different recorded values.
- Each step up the scale of one unit is of equal size. E.g. the difference between pressures of 80 and 81 mmHg is exactly the same as that between 94 and 95 mmHg.

2.2.1 Continuous Measured Data – Normal and Non-Normal Distribution

Continuous measured data needs to be further subdivided according to whether it follows a normal distribution or not, as many statistical methods will only work with normally distributed data. Non-normal data needs alternative approaches. It is best to avoid statistical tests for normality (Kolmogorov–Smirnov, Anderson–Darling etc.) as the results are easily misinterpreted (See Rowe 2015, Chapter 4).[1] However, there are a number of different approaches to determining whether your data is normally distributed or not.

Whether data is or is not normally distributed is most easily decided by preparing a histogram of the data. Unless your sample sizes are very large, group your results into a small number of bars as you only want to check the general shape of the distribution. Figure 2.1a shows an example of normally distributed data. This is commonly referred to as a "bell-shaped" distribution and it has three features:

- The greatest frequencies (tallest histogram bars) are somewhere near the middle of the range of values observed. What we **do not** want is to see is the tallest histogram bars at either the far left or right hand end of the horizontal scale (as shown in Figure 2.1b).
- The results are all clustered around a single point; they **do not** fall into two distinct groups of high and low values (as shown in Figure 2.1c). Normally distributed data is said to be "Unimodal."
- For both low and high values, frequencies decline steadily toward zero with no sudden cut-off (as shown in Figure 2.1d).

---

[1] Rowe P. Essential statistics for the pharmaceutical sciences, 2nd edn. Chichester: Wiley, 2015.

Figure 2.1b shows a common form of non-normality. The majority of individuals are clustered at the low end of the scale, and there is a long tail of high values. This is referred to as "Positive skew."

Figure 2.1c shows a further form of non-normality – bimodality. The data forms two distinct clusters of low and high values. (The term "Poymodality" applies to any case with more than one cluster of values.)

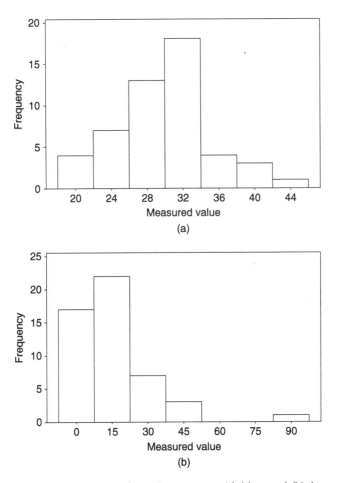

Figure 2.1 A continuously varying measure with (a) normal, (b) skewed, and (c) bimodal distribution. In (d) the highest and lowest values (tails) from an otherwise normal distribution are missing.

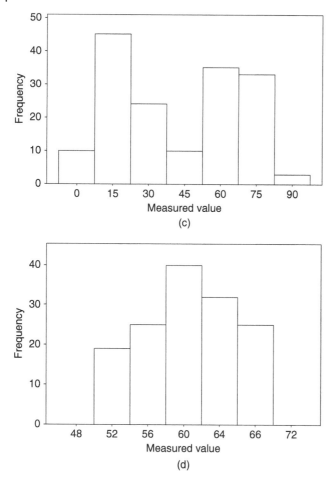

Figure 2.1 *(Continued)*

Figure 2.1d shows a final form of non-normality. Results are cut off suddenly at values of around 50 and 70; for a true normal distribution, there should be a more gradual decline in frequencies beyond these limits.

NOTE: Do not expect to get ideal bell-shaped distributions, especially with small samples. The distribution shown in Figure 2.1a is perfectly acceptable. We just don't want to see obvious deviations from normality such as seen in Figure 2.1b, c, or d.

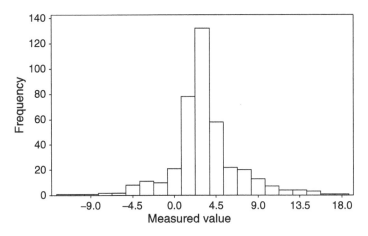

Figure 2.2 Histogram of "Long-tailed" data, i.e. data that includes both low and high outlying values.

The only important deviation from normality that is not easily detected from a histogram is where there are outlying extreme values in both the low and high tail (Referred to as "Long-tailed" distributions). Figure 2.2 shows data that suffers this problem, but this form of non-normality is not always easy to diagnose from a histogram, and an alternative method is required. The next paragraph shows how this problem can be detected.

To detect whether your data has a long-tailed distribution, it is useful to produce a "normal probability plot," which uses the mean and standard deviation (SD) of the sample and looks for any differences between the data distribution that would be expected for a normal distribution and what you actually observe (the video mentioned at the end of the chapter shows how to produce these plots). An ideal line where all points should fall is usually added to the graph by the software. Figure 2.3a shows such a plot for a set of data that is almost exactly normally distributed; all the points are very close to the line of perfect fit for normality. Figure 2.3b shows a plot for a long-tailed distribution. The points for the lowest values are all displaced to the left of the ideal line, i.e. these values are markedly lower than they should be for a true normal distribution ("low outliers"). At the other end of the scale, the highest points are to the right of the ideal line (values that are higher than they ought to be – "high outliers"). If your

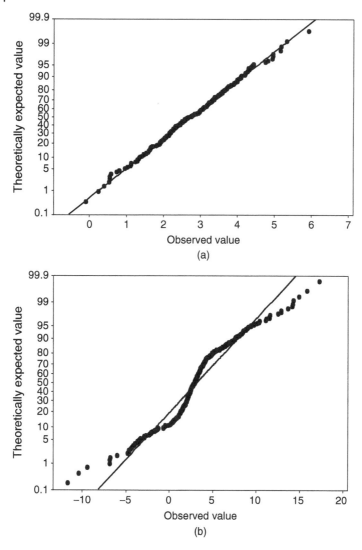

Figure 2.3 Normal probability plots of (a) normally distributed data and (b) long-tailed data.

data produces a normal probability plot like that shown in Figure 2.3b, then you should treat your data as non-normal. In further chapters that discuss methods requiring normality, you will be advised how to handle non-normality.

See the video listed at the end of the chapter for details of using a statistical package to check data normality.

2.2.2   Transforming Non-Normal Data

When data is not normally distributed, it may be possible to manipulate it to bring it closer to normality. This is referred to as "data transformation."

- Data showing positive skew (as in Figure 2.1b) can often be returned to normality by a technique called "Log transformation." A video listed at the end of this chapter gives practical details.
- Data showing bimodality, severe absence of tails, or long tails (Figures 2.1c and d and 2.2) cannot easily be transformed to normality.

Rowe (2015) Chapters 4 and 21 gives further details on non-normal distributions and their transformation to normality.

2.3   Ordinal Data

Here, the characteristic to be measured is often subjective in nature. For example, we might assess how patients feel about a treatment they have received, using a score, of (say) one to five with the following equivalences:

1 = Strongly dissatisfied
2 = Somewhat dissatisfied
3 = Neither satisfied nor dissatisfied
4 = Generally satisfied
5 = Very satisfied

The data consists of categorizations, but the important thing is that the categories have a natural order to them. There is a definite ranking from "Strongly dissatisfied" to "Very satisfied" via three intermediate grades.

This type of data has the following characteristics:

- It is discontinuous. Only these five integer values are available. There are no scores of 1.45 or any other fractional value.
- Ordinal scales usually allow only small numbers of possible values (five in the current case).

- It often cannot be assumed that all the steps up the scale are of equal significance. Although you may have scored gradings as 1,2,3 etc., you cannot assume that the difference between "Strongly dissatisfied" and "Somewhat dissatisfied" is of exactly the same importance as that between "Somewhat dissatisfied" and "Neither satisfied nor dissatisfied."

2.4 Categorical Data

This is also known as "Nominal" data. Here there is no intention to *measure* a characteristic: we are just categorizing. For example, advice might be provided by nurses, pharmacists, or physiotherapists. These do not form any sort of scale; they are just three different professions. Frequently there are just two options, obvious cases being Male/Female, Yes/No or Successful/Failed; these are referred to as "Binary" or "Dichotomous."

2.5 Ambiguous Cases

There are a couple of problematic areas where things are not as obvious as in the examples given above.

2.5.1 A Continuously Varying Measure that has been Divided into a Small Number of Ranges

If you use subjects' ages to divide them into two groups ("Younger" and "Older"), then with just two ranges, your data clearly become simple, categorical (Nominal) data. However, with three ranges (e.g. "Younger," "Middle aged," and "Older"), you could either view these as categorical or consider that you have created an ordinal scale of measurement. Your decision, in terms of statistical analysis, will depend on what sort of relationship you are exploring with the data.

- If you are investigating the relationship between age and the likelihood of a degenerative disease, you might want to test for a simple trend where greater age is associated with greater risk of the condition. The model being tested would be that the risk of the condition increases as we go from Younger to Middle aged and then there would be a further increase as we pass from Middle aged to Older. Here, you should treat age as an ordinal measurement. Such relationships are referred to as "Monotonic"; as one measure (age) increases, the other one (e.g. likelihood of an age-related disease) either consistently increases or consistently decreases; it would not increase as we pass from the Younger group to those who are Middle aged but then go down again among those who are Older.

- However, in other cases (such as linking age to ability to perform a particular task), you may need to allow for the possibility of a more complex relationship with age. Ability might be low among the young and inexperienced, higher in later years, but then lower again in old age, owing to degeneration of some physical or cognitive feature. Here, the relationship is not necessarily monotonic, and it would be best to treat the age groups as just a series of categories, in order to allow for any pattern of change in aptitude with age.

2.5.2 Composite Scores with a Wide Range of Possible Values

In surveys, or clinical assessments, we frequently meet methods where an overall indicator is obtained by adding up the scores obtained on a number of questions. The results are technically discontinuous – no fractional scores can arise – so maybe we should treat it as ordinal. However, there may be such a wide range of possible values that it becomes effectively continuously varying. An example is the Hamilton Depression Rating Scale, which sums the scores from seventeen (or more) questions, producing a wide range of possible values. The large number of allowable values may also allow a normal distribution to develop, and it is reasonable to treat such data as continuous measured values. If you are using a composite score approach based on a series of questions that you have designed, you should look at Chapter 20 – Cronbach's Alpha.

2.6   Relevant Videos etc.

The following are available at
www.wiley.com/go/Mackridge/APracticalApproachtoUsingStatisticsin
HealthResearch

Videos

Video_1.1_SPSS_Basics: The absolute basics of using SPSS.

Video_2.1_NormalityTesting: Using SPSS to determine whether measured data follows a normal distribution and log transformation to improve normality.

3

Presenting and Summarizing Data

It is often useful to describe a whole data set in a single graph or summary statistic. However, there are no universal solutions to doing this – the best way to describe a data set will depend on a number of things, particularly what you are hoping to show with the data. Firstly, you need to identify the type of data you have collected (continuous measured, ordinal, or categorical – see Chapter 2), and then you will need to explore the options in order to find an approach that honestly and clearly illustrates the key features of your particular data set.

3.1   Continuous Measured Data

For a full description of measurement data, you need to indicate how great the values are and also how much variability there is within the data set. For the former, you will use measures such as the mean or median. For variability, you will most likely use the standard deviation (SD).

Before you start generating descriptive statistics, you should first explore the data graphically. A graph may well reveal that your data has an awkward distribution that requires a careful choice of descriptors. The distribution of the data can usually be best illustrated using a histogram,[1] but with small data sets, these can be misleading; even if a particular

---

[1] Note that histograms are distinct from bar charts. Histograms use data that was originally on a continuously varying scale, but we have collected the values into a series of ranges. To reflect the fact that the data were originally continuous, the bars are drawn with no gaps between them.

A Practical Approach to Using Statistics in Health Research: From Planning to Reporting, First Edition. Adam Mackridge and Philip Rowe.
© 2018 John Wiley & Sons, Inc. Published 2018 by John Wiley & Sons, Inc.
Companion website: www.wiley.com/go/Mackridge/
APracticalApproachtoUsingStatisticsinHealthResearch

outcome is normally distributed, a small sample will most likely fail to generate a histogram that looks remotely like the ideal bell-shaped distribution. For these small samples, a dot plot may be more useful.

Rowe (2015, Chapter 3)[2] gives a detailed description of methods to summarize continuous measured data. These are summarized below.

3.1.1 Normally Distributed Data – Using the Mean and Standard Deviation

If, when you have plotted your data graphically, the results reasonably approximate a normal distribution, the mean and standard deviation (SD) are likely to be the best summary statistics. Any mean value that is key to the conclusions you draw should be accompanied by a 95% confidence interval so that the reader can appreciate the likely degree of precision of your result in describing the population from which your sample was drawn. The only real exception to this rule is where the value you report is not intended to be a sample estimate of some underlying population value. For example, you might report the mean age of the subjects in your study group. This is simply a description of your sample and is not intended to estimate the mean age of some larger population; no confidence interval is required. See the videos listed at the end of this chapter for details of using statistical packages to generate descriptive statistics and confidence intervals.

3.1.2 Data With Outliers, e.g. Skewed Data – Using Quartiles and the Median

Data sets for outcomes that cannot take negative values (e.g. blood urea concentration) may not contain low outliers (values far below the mean) as there is a natural lower limit to the data distribution at zero. However, there may be values way above the mean (high outliers). The resultant distribution is said to suffer "Positive skew" (See Figure 2.1a). With skewed data, high outlying values can disproportionately affect your calculations, leading to a mean that fails to represent the bulk of the data. Quartile based indicators (See below) may be more appropriate.

---

[2] Rowe P. Essential statistics for the pharmaceutical sciences, 2nd edn. Chichester: Wiley, 2015.

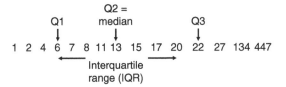

Mean = 48.9
SD   = 114.8

Figure 3.1 The quartiles for a data set with ranked values ranging from 1 to 447. The quartiles, median, and interquartile range (IQR) are indicated. The mean and SD are also included.

Quartiles are values that lie one quarter, half, and then three quarters of the way up a set of data that has been ranked (all data are listed from the smallest to the largest). The median is simply another name for the second quartile: it has 50% of the observations above and 50% below it. It acts as an alternative indicator of central tendency that can replace the mean.

Figure 3.1 shows the quartiles (Q1, Q2, and Q3) for a ranked data set. The three quartile points are selected so that there are equal numbers of observations below Q1, between Q1 and Q2, between Q2 and Q3 and above Q3. In the current case, there are three observations between each of the quartile values. The quartile values are Q1 = 6, Q2 = 13, and Q3 = 22. The median from Figure 3.1 is 13.

The data set includes two high outlying values (134 and 447). The presence of these inflates the mean to 48.9. The mean would provide a poor description of the dataset. It is not representative: all but two of the values are considerably lower. In a similar way, the SD (±114.8) is inordinately affected by the two outliers.

The interquartile range (IQR) fulfills a role similar to that of the SD. It is the difference between the first and third quartiles. The greater the range of values in your data set (i.e. the more spread out it is), the greater the IQR will be. It therefore acts as a measure of data variability. The IQR is 16 (6 to 22).

In contrast to the mean, the median is relatively unaffected by the outliers, and its value (13) is much more typical and representative of the data set as a whole. Likewise, the IQR is largely immune to the effect of outliers. This ability of the median and IQR to resist the effects of a few atypical results leads them to be described as "Robust," whereas the mean and SD are not considered robust. Where a data set contains outliers (e.g. positively skewed data), the median and IQR are likely to be the most appropriate descriptors.

See the end of this chapter for a video showing how to obtain quartile values.

3.1.3   Polymodal Data – Using the Modes

It does not happen very often, but occasionally data may break up into two (or more) distinct clusters of high and low values. Figure 3.2 shows a histogram of body temperatures among a group of individuals who had been exposed to the common cold virus. Although they are not fully separated, there is a strong suggestion of two sub-groups, with lower and higher temperatures – a likely explanation being that some have caught the virus while others have resisted it. The mean temperature for the whole group is 37.1°C, but this does not provide a good description of the situation as it falls in the gap between the two peaks.

The data in Figure 3.2 is "Bimodal" and the summary description of the data must reflect that fact. This can be achieved by reporting the modes for the two sub-groups. The modes are simply the values with peak frequencies – in this case 36.6 and 37.4°C.

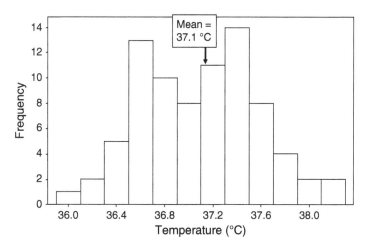

Figure 3.2 Histogram of body temperatures among individuals exposed to the common cold virus.

3.2   Ordinal Data

3.2.1   Ordinal Scales With a Narrow Range of Possible Values

The first thing you should always do with ordinal data recorded on scales that allow only a limited range of values (e.g. five point Likert items) is report the number (and possibly proportion) of individuals recorded as having each possible value. If a value on the scale has a frequency of zero, this information should be included. This information can be presented either numerically or in a bar chart.[3] Whatever method of data presentation is used, it must include the counts (not just the proportions) for each value. A bar chart (Figure 3.3) has been used to present scores for opinions on a new appointment booking system.

Taking a further step, you may want to produce a summary statistic to represent your ordinal data. Summary statistics are likely to be especially

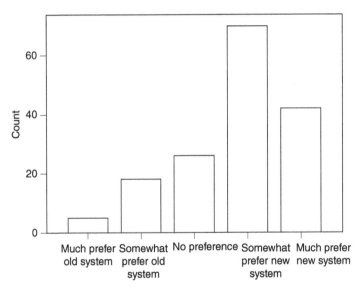

Figure 3.3 Bar chart of opinions concerning changes to an appointment booking system.

---

[3] Ordinal data consists of a series of distinct categories, so graphs should be bar charts and not histograms (i.e. the bars should have spaces between them).

useful where you need to compare two sets of ordinal data. The median and IQR are the most widely used/accepted statistics for this purpose, and it is best to try these as they are uncontroversial and unlikely to lead to problems getting work published. However, with scales that allow only a small number of possible values, the median can be very insensitive and may fail to illustrate key aspects of your data. In such cases, it may be appropriate to also report the mean and explain that the mean has been included because the median was too insensitive.

Appendix 1 to this chapter provides an example where the median fails to reflect the difference between two sets of ordinal data and the additional use of the mean would be useful.

3.2.2   Ordinal Scales With a Wide Range of Possible Values

With scales that allow a wide range of possible values, you would not report the number of individuals having each of the possible values, but a bar chart may be a useful way to convey the distribution of ranges of scores (e.g. 1–5, 6–10, 11–15 etc.)

Describing the central tendency of wide ranging scales is less problematic than with the narrow-range scales, and quoting the median plus IQR works well in many cases. The insensitivity problem mentioned in section 3.2.1 is much less troublesome, although it may still raise its ugly head where large numbers of respondents opt for values near the middle of the scale and avoid the extremes. If this problem arises then it is best to adopt the solution described in Section 3.2.1 quote the median, point out its shortcomings, and use this to justify the additional use of the mean.

If you are using a well-established scale such as the Hamilton Depression Rating scale or Alcohol Use Disorders Identification Test (AUDIT), check the literature to see what statistics (median plus IQR or mean plus SD) are commonly used with that particular scale. If you go with the herd, (a) nobody is likely to object and (b) your results will be directly comparable with those already published.

3.2.3   Dividing an Ordinal Scale Into a Small Number of Ranges (e.g. Satisfactory/Unsatisfactory or Poor/Acceptable/Good)

In some cases, e.g. the AUDIT alcohol risk scale, wide ranging scores may be categorized into a smaller number of clinically meaningful groups (for AUDIT: Low risk; Increasing risk; High Risk; Dependent). In such cases, you may decide to present your results in the form of numbers in each macro-group. This can be done numerically or in a bar chart.

Some caution is needed when using this approach within comparative studies. Aggregating the data into a small number of ranges may be a useful way to illustrate the difference between two groups, but if you need to perform a statistical test, you may find that the process of aggregation destroys a lot of information. For example, your original data might be collected using a six point Likert item, which could then be converted into two categories such as "satisfactory" and "unsatisfactory." However, you may find that while a statistical test on the six point ordinal data achieves statistical significance, the same data expressed as two categories is non-significant.

3.2.4 Summary for Ordinal Data

Presenting data:

- For narrow-range scales, always report the number (and possibly the proportion) of individuals recorded as having each value on the scale. This could be done numerically or as a bar chart.
- For wider ranging scales, a bar chart may be useful, but do not report the numbers in each individual category. It may be appropriate in some cases to create much smaller numbers of categories arising from the "scores," such as in the case of AUDIT, and present these numerically or in a bar chart.

Using summary statistics:

- It is usually most appropriate to illustrate the key aspects of the data using the median and IQR, but if this approach is too insensitive, the mean and SD may also be required. If you use the mean, also quote the median, and explain why the additional use of the mean was necessary.
- If there is established custom and practice in your area of research or for a particular validated scale, go with the flow.

3.3 Categorical Data

Categorical data is described in terms of the numbers and proportions of individual cases that fall into each category. Proportions will probably be expressed as percentages, but the actual counts must also be provided for clarity and openness in reporting. Key outcomes that are to be expressed as proportions should always be accompanied by a 95% confidence interval (CI), so that the reader will be aware of the uncertainty associated with random sampling error. For example, you might report that "Of the 234 participants, 129 (55%; 95% CI 49 to 61%) preferred to see a doctor rather than a nurse."

When presenting proportions graphically, it is important that the reader also has access to the actual numbers in each group, either through annotation on the chart itself, or separately in the related text. Proportions can be shown as either bar charts or pie charts, but the latter are often viewed negatively in academic circles as it is often harder to see patterns in the data, and a bar chart can be used to present two sets of data side by side to illustrate differences between different conditions. Under no circumstances use pie charts with only two categories – they are of no value whatsoever.

3.4   Relevant Videos etc.

The following are available at
www.wiley.com/go/Mackridge/APracticalApproachtoUsingStatisticsin
HealthResearch

Videos

Video_1.1_SPSS_Basics: The absolute basics of using SPSS.
Video_3.1_Descriptives Proportions: Using SPSS to obtain the mean, 95% confidence interval for the mean, standard deviation, quartiles, and the median and proportions for categorized data.

Appendix 1: An Example of the Insensitivity of the Median When Used to Describe Data from an Ordinal Scale With a Narrow Range of Possible Values

This example concerns a Likert item asking about agreement with the statement that "I would be happy to book future appointments electronically." The grading scale is 1=Strongly disagree; 2=Disagree; 3=Neutral; 4=Agree; 5=Strongly agree. We have compared the opinions of patients aged under 50 years versus those 50 or over. There are 45 patients in each study group. The results are shown in Table 3.1 and the medians (middle ranking individuals) are emphasized.

Table 3.1 Levels of agreement among younger and older patients with the statement that "I would be happy to book future appointments electronically." Higher values reflect stronger agreement. Medians are emboldened.

Under fifty years:
1 1 2 2 3 3 3 3 3 3 3 3 3 3 3 3 3 3 3 3 3 3 3 3 **3** 3 3 4 4 4 4 4 4 4 4 4 4 4 5 5 5 5 5 5 5 5 5
Fifty years plus:
1 1 1 1 1 1 1 1 1 2 2 2 2 2 2 2 2 2 3 3 3 3 **3** 3 3 3 3 3 3 3 3 3 3 3 3 3 3 3 3 3 3 3 4 4 5

Mean values: Younger 3.51; Older 2.48
Median values: Younger 3; Older 3

Among the younger participants, many are supportive (scores of four or five) with relatively few opposed (scoring one or two). With the older individuals, we have the opposite pattern – plenty of opposition and not much support. However, the median scores fail to reflect this trend: for both groups it is three. In contrast, the mean values (3.51 and 2.48) successfully illustrate the difference between the age groups.

4

Choosing a Statistical Test

In this chapter, you are walked through a series of steps, by the end of which you should have identified the key characteristics of your study. There are checklists (please download a copy from the companion website – see the end of this chapter) that you can fill in as you work through the chapter. These will ensure you have a complete list of characteristics to help you select the most appropriate statistical test for your study.

This chapter may seem dauntingly long but, for any given study, you will only need to read the relevant sections; you will be guided to skip past many parts.

4.1   Identify the Factor and Outcome

Statistical tests are usually used when we suspect that there may be some form of cause and effect relationship.[1] Translating this into "stat speak," there is an "Outcome" that may be influenced by a "Factor."

- Factor = Cause
- Outcome = Effect

Factor–outcome relationships may arise from an active intervention (such as treating a disease with a particular drug) or from an existing

---

[1] It is important to note that, in most cases, statistical testing will only assess the strength of a *relationship* between a factor and an outcome and does **not** assess whether the factor has any *causative* action on the outcome. See section 6.8 for more information.

A Practical Approach to Using Statistics in Health Research: From Planning to Reporting, First Edition. Adam Mackridge and Philip Rowe.
Companion website: www.wiley.com/go/Mackridge/
APracticalApproachtoUsingStatisticsinHealthResearch

Table 4.1 Examples of factors and outcomes.

	Description	Factor	Outcome
Active intervention	1) Compare effectiveness of advice plus provision of nicotine patches *versus* advice alone on smoking cessation	Provision or non-provision of nicotine patches	Do or do not smoke any cigarettes for the next twelve weeks.
	2) Compare the perceived clarity of an old, and two new, versions of an advisory leaflet	Old version or first/second new version has been read	Perceived clarity of the three leaflets (Scored 0-4)
	3) Compare cholesterol levels in a group who continue to use butter versus a group who change to a cholesterol lowering spread	Used butter or cholesterol lowering spread	Cholesterol levels at the end of the period of the study
	4) Is daily dosage of an ACE inhibitor linked to the likelihood of a dry cough?	Daily dose of ACE inhibitor	Presence or absence of cough
Existing characteristic	5) Does participant sex affect likelihood of retention in a methadone maintenance program?	Male or female	Is or is not retained in the program at twelve weeks
	6) Do post code areas with high or low levels of social deprivation show different levels of alcohol consumption?	Area has high or low level of deprivation	Average per capita alcohol consumption in each area
	7) Are there differences between the scores on a knowledge test concerning infection control for doctors, nurses, and ancillary staff	Professional group: doctor, nurse, or ancillary staff	Score on the test (scores on a scale of zero to five)
	8) Is lung function affected by the distance that children walk to school in an urban area with severe vehicular air pollution?	Distance walked	FEV1 (Forced Expiratory Volume in one second)
	9) Does length of hospital stay increase risk of acquiring an infection	Number of days admitted to hospital	Acquisition of infection (Yes/No)

characteristic (such as the sex of a participant). Some examples of possible studies and the factors and outcomes that would be involved are shown in Table 4.1

Your first job is to identify the factor and outcome that you plan to investigate.

> Identify the factor and outcome that you wish to study and complete line A of Checklist 1 (Copy available at end of Section 4.2).

4.2 Identify the Type of Data Used to Record the Relevant Factor

Next you need to determine the type of data that you will use to record your factor. See Chapter 2 for more information on data types.

In all the examples above (except numbers 4, 8, and 9), the factor would be recorded as categorical data. For example, in case one, nicotine patches were *provided* or *not provided* and in case seven, profession is *doctor, nurse,* or *ancillary staff.*

In examples 4, 8, and 9, the factor would be recorded as a continuous measurement (size of daily dose, distance walked, or number of days).

> Identify the type of data that would be used to record the relevant **factor** and enter this onto line B of Checklist 1.

First check list for identification of appropriate statistical test

Checklist 1 *(All study types)*				
A	**Identify factor and outcome**	Factor =		Outcome =
B	**Data type for factor?**	☐ Categorical	☐ Ordinal	☐ Continuous measured

If your factor is of a measured type (ordinal or continuous measured), then jump to Section 4.4 (Correlation and regression). If it is categorical, then continue with Section 4.3.

4.3   Statistical Methods Where the Factor is Categorical

4.3.1   Identify the Type of Data Used to Record the Outcome

Again, see Chapter 2 for more information on data types.

- **Continuous measured (or "scale")**: From Table 4.1, examples 3 and 6, concerning cholesterol levels (measured in mmol/L or mg/dL) and alcohol consumption (units of alcohol per day) both have a continuous measured outcome.
- **Ordinal**: In example 2, the measure of leaflet clarity is ordinal as it can take only a small number of possible values (0–4), and these form an ordered scale. Similarly, with example 7, the knowledge scores are ordinal.
- **Categorical (or "nominal")**: Examples 1 and 5 (cigarette avoidance and participants remaining within a methadone maintenance program) have categorical outcomes.

> Identify what type of **outcome** data you are analysing, and complete line C of Checklist 2 (Copy available at end of Section **4.3.4**).

4.3.2   Is Continuous Measured Outcome Data Normally Distributed or Can It Be Transformed to Normality?

You only need to complete this stage if your outcome data is of the continuous measured type – if your outcome data is ordinal or categorical, go to Section **4.3.3**.

You need to assess whether your measured data approximates a normal distribution. Sections 2.2.1 and 2.2.2, and the relevant video, describe the process for assessing normality and transformation to normality.

There are three possible conclusions. Your data may be:

- **Normally distributed**, or a reasonable approximation to this: analyze your data as a continuous measured outcome.
- **Not** normally distributed, but **can** be transformed to approximate normality (see Section 2.2.2 for more information on how to do this): analyze your transformed data as a continuous measured outcome.
- **Not** normal and **cannot** be successfully transformed: treat your outcome data as if it were ordinal.

> If outcome was initially recorded as continuous measured data, decide whether (with or without transformation) it can be confirmed as continuous measured or should be treated as if it were ordinal. If necessary, modify line C in Checklist 2.

4.3.3 Identify Whether Your Sets of Outcome Data Are Related or Independent

There are two ways to perform a comparative study. These result in outcome data being "Related" or "Independent."

Related data sets

You could design an investigation in which a single group of individuals (or institutions) are studied under one set of conditions and then study the same group under altered conditions, each individual being studied twice. In the third example in Table 4.1, you could study all participants while using butter and record their cholesterol levels, then transfer them all to a cholesterol lowering spread and re-measure their cholesterol levels. Each participant would thus generate two outcome results. The data would then consist of related pairs of observations (two from the first patient, two from the next, and so on). This is referred to as *related* data. (The alternative terms "Dependent" or "Paired" may also be used.)

There may be more than two data sets to be compared, but the outcome can still be related. In the case of the advisory leaflet (example 2 in Table 4.1), there is an old version and two different, updated versions, giving a three-way comparison. If you were to have each participant assess all three leaflets, this would generate three sets of related data.

The most common reason why results are considered to be related is that two or more observations are from the same person. That is true for all the examples given so far. However, there are other causes for data being considered as related. For example, you might use matched pairs of participants, i.e. pairs of people chosen as having similar demographics – almost certainly of similar age and gender, and perhaps matched on other characteristics. Within each pair, one participant might receive an active treatment with the other getting a placebo. This will lead to a data structure containing pairs of related observations.

Independent data sets

Alternatively, you could design a study whereby one group of participants experience one set of conditions and another separate group experience different conditions, each individual being studied once only. For the butter/spread study, you could split the participants into two separate groups. All those in one group would use butter with those in the other group using the cholesterol lowering spread. Each participant would now contribute just one observation and that observation stands alone – independent of any other. This is "*Independent*" data. (The alternative term "Unpaired" may be used.)

In the case of the advisory leaflet (example 2 in Table 4.1), if you were to split the participants into three groups and have individuals in each group review only one leaflet each, this would give three sets of independent data.

> Identify whether the structure of your outcome data is related or independent. Complete line D of Checklist 2.

4.3.4 For the Factor, How Many Levels Are Being Studied?

In examples 1, 3, 5, and 6 in Table 4.1, you would compare two sets of data against each other, but examples 2 and 7 involve three-way comparisons. The number of study groups to be compared are commonly referred to as "Levels." Thus, in most of the examples in Table 4.1, the factor has two levels, but the studies on advisory leaflets or professional groups have three levels.

> Identify the number of levels for the factor to be studied. Complete line E of Checklist 2.

	Checklist 2 *(Studies with **categorical** factors only)*		
C	**Data type for outcome?**	☐ Categorical	☐ Ordinal	☐ Continuous measured
D	**Outcome data is independent or related?**	☐ Independent		☐ Related
E	**How many levels for the factor?**	☐ Two		☐ More than two

4.3.5 Determine the Appropriate Statistical Method for Studies with a Categorical Factor

Using the information from completed Checklist 2, select the appropriate method from Table 4.2. You do not need to read any more of this chapter.

Table 4.2 Identification of appropriate statistical tests for studies with a categorical factor.

	Independent (Unpaired) data			Related (Dependent/ Paired) data		
	Continuous measured outcome	**Ordinal outcome**	**Categorical outcome**	**Continuous measured outcome**	**Ordinal outcome**	**Categorical outcome**
Two levels	Two-sample t-test	Mann–Whitney test	Contingency chi-square test	Paired t-test	Wilcoxon paired samples test	McNemar's test
More than two levels	One-way analysis of variance	Kruskal–Wallis test	Contingency chi-square test	Repeated measures analysis of variance	Friedman test	No test appropriate for this book's intended readership

4.4   Correlation and Regression with a Measured Factor

The rest of this chapter is only relevant if your **factor** consists of some form of measured data (continuous measured or ordinal).

4.4.1   What Type of Data Was Used to Record Your Factor and Outcome?

You first need to identify whether your measured factor would be recorded as ordinal or continuous measured data and whether your outcome is categorical, ordinal, or continuous measured. In Table 4.1, examples 4, 8, and 9 all involve a *factor* that is a continuous measurement. In examples 4 and 9, the *outcome* is categorical and in example 8 it is a continuous measurement.

> Identify what type of **factor** and **outcome** data you are analysing and complete lines F and G of Checklist 3.

	Checklist 3 *(Studies with **ordinal or continuous measured** factors)*			
F	**Data type for factor?**	☐ Ordinal		☐ Continuous measured
G	**Data type for outcome?**	☐ Categorical	☐ Ordinal	☐ Continuous measured

Unless both your factor and outcome are continuous measurements, Table 4.3 will guide you toward correlation or regression techniques, which are covered in Chapters 17 to 19, and you do not need to read any more of this chapter.

If both factor and outcome are continuous measurements, proceed to Section **4.4.2**.

4.4.2   When Both the Factor and the Outcome Consist of Continuous Measured Values, Select Between Pearson and Spearman Correlation

There are two forms of correlation that may be appropriate: "Pearson" and "Spearman." The former is used so widely that it is often referred

Table 4.3 Selection of correlation or regression techniques depending on type of data used to record the factor and outcome.

	Factor	
Outcome	**Ordinal**	**Continuous measured**
Categorical	Logistic regression	Logistic regression
Ordinal	Spearman correlation	Spearman correlation
Continuous measured	Spearman correlation	Read Section 4.4.2 to choose between Pearson or Spearman correlation

to simply as "Correlation" without further clarification. Broadly speaking, you should use Pearson correlation when it is appropriate, as it is somewhat more powerful than the Spearman version. However, Spearman correlation is non-parametric and consequently more robust than the Pearson form, so there are various problematic data sets where Spearman is preferable. The potential problems are described below.

When both the factor and the outcome are continuously measured, it is important to inspect a scatter plot and compare it to Figures 4.1 to 4.5 to identify which type of relationship it most closely approximates.

Figure 4.1 shows two forms of relationship where (a) the Y value rises steadily as X increases or (b) falls steadily as X increases. Either

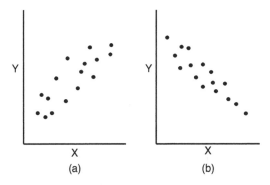

(a) (b)

Figure 4.1 Approximately linear relationship – (a) positive correlation and (b) negative correlation.

of these is ideally suited to a Pearson correlation assessment to evaluate the strength of the relationship.

Figure 4.2 shows a cluster of points and an outlying value. Pearson correlation is rather sensitive to a small number of outliers, which can result in a misleadingly high value for the correlation coefficient. As such, Spearman correlation should be used as it is more robust and will be much less influenced by outliers

> Check whether there are strong outliers and complete line H of Checklist 4 (Copy near end of Section 4.4).

In Figure 4.3a, Y first increases and then decreases, as the X value increases. In part b, the value for Y falls initially, then rises. These are in contrast to Figures 4.1.1a or b, where Y consistently increases or

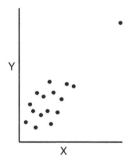

Figure 4.2 A cluster of points with outlier(s).

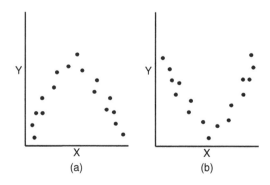

(a)   (b)

Figure 4.3 Relationships that are clearly not monotonic.

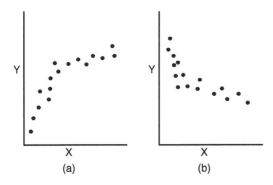

Figure 4.4 Monotonic, but clearly non-linear relationships – (a) positive and (b) negative.

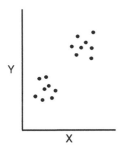

Figure 4.5 Data with distinct clusters.

consistently decreases. Relationships such as those in Figure 4.1 are described as "Monotonic," whereas those in 4.3 are not.

In Figure 4.4, throughout both graphs, there is a consistent trend, either always upwards or always downwards, so the relationships are monotonic; however, the relationships have a definite curvature: they are non-linear.

> Determine whether the relationship is monotonic and whether it is approximately linear. Complete lines I and J of Checklist 4.

Figure 4.5 shows a case that would generate a high value for either the Pearson or Spearman correlation coefficients and which would apparently provide statistically significant evidence of correlation. However, the reality is that there are two sub-populations with differing properties. No form of correlation would be usefully applicable to such data. It may be possible to identify a characteristic that distinguishes these two groups (e.g. participant sex), and you could separate the data thus into two sub-sets. You could then conduct a correlation analysis within each sub-set to determine if there are relationships between the factor and outcome. However, you should be clear in your reporting that this analysis was secondary to that which you planned prior to data collection (see Chapter 5 for more details).

Check for clearly distinct clusters and complete line K of Checklist 4.

Checklist 4 *(Studies where both the **factor and the outcome are continuous measured data**)*	
H	☐ No data outliers	☐ Data outliers
I	☐ Monotonic	☐ Not monotonic
J	☐ Approximately linear	☐ Clearly non-linear
K	☐ No distinct data clusters	☐ Distinct data clusters

With Checklist 4 completed, you should now know whether your data passes four tests and you can determine the way forward:

- All four tests satisfactory (no clear outliers, relationship is monotonic and approximately linear with no distinct clusters) – Use Pearson correlation.
- The relationship is monotonic **and** does not have distinct clusters, but there are outliers and/or the relationship is clearly non-linear – Use Spearman correlation.
- There are distinct clusters and/or the relationship is not monotonic – no form of correlation is appropriate.

If the data forms distinct clusters (as in Figure 4.5), then it would be useful to investigate what differentiates the two (or more) groups (see above).

4.5   Relevant Additional Material

The following are available at
www.wiley.com/go/Mackridge/APracticalApproachtoUsingStatisticsin
HealthResearch
Companion checklist: Checklist for identification of study characteristics and selection of statistical analyses.

5

Multiple Testing

5.1   What Is Multiple Testing and Why Does It Matter?

In a typical simple study, you would look at the impact of one factor on one outcome. Let us imagine you find yourself investigating whether children raised in vegetarian families are more, or less, likely to develop a skin condition compared to children raised on an omnivorous diet, and also assume that diet type actually has absolutely no real effect on the risk of this condition. If you analyzed your data in the conventional way, requiring a P-value of less than 0.05, you will have 95% assurance of correctly arriving at a conclusion of non-significance.

However, there is still that residual 5% risk that random error has created results that, incorrectly, indicate a difference between the groups, with a P-value below 0.05 leading you to falsely claim that diet does have an effect. Such an event is termed a "False positive." The risk of this happening is always present, but traditionally we consider the 5% risk small enough to be tolerable.

If you had restricted yourself to looking only at diet, the risk level would remain where it is supposed to be, i.e. 5%. However, if you wanted to look at multiple factors affecting your primary outcome, you might have recorded other details about each child, such as gender, ethnicity, and residential area (inner city/suburban/rural), and we will also assume that none of these have any real influence upon the condition. You could then run tests for each of the factor/outcome pairs, which is what we mean by multiple testing. When you carry out

A Practical Approach to Using Statistics in Health Research: From Planning to Reporting, First Edition. Adam Mackridge and Philip Rowe.
© 2018 John Wiley & Sons, Inc. Published 2018 by John Wiley & Sons, Inc.
Companion website: www.wiley.com/go/Mackridge/
APracticalApproachtoUsingStatisticsinHealthResearch

four tests, each one would generate a 5% risk of a false positive, giving something approaching a 20% risk of at least one false positive. A 5% risk may be tolerable, but 20% is not. Likewise, you might be looking at multiple outcomes for a given factor, and the same issue would be present.

5.2 What Can We Do to Avoid an Excessive Risk of False Positives?

If you have followed the general philosophy of this book and kept to a simple design – one factor influencing one outcome – then multiple testing will not arise. This is one of the reasons why it is desirable to select one factor and one outcome for the design of your study – to make your findings easy to interpret. However, in the real world, some complexity may raise its ugly head. There are several possible solutions:

5.2.1 Use of Omnibus Tests

If you were planning to study residential area as a possible factor affecting the risk of a skin condition, you might produce three study groups (inner city, suburban, and rural). In such a case, there is no need or justification for comparing every possible pair of groups sequentially and thereby performing three separate tests. Whatever type of outcome data you have collected – continuous measured, ordinal, or categorical – there is a suitable procedure – One way analysis of variance, Kruskal–Wallis test, or Chi-square test respectively – that can consider all the groups within a single analysis. This approach does not constitute multiple testing, as only one test is used. Where the omnibus test is significant, you may then want to look in more detail at exactly which group differs from which other. In the individual chapters on these methods, there are instructions for doing this without raising the risk of false positives.

5.2.2 Distinguishing Between Primary and Secondary/ Exploratory Analyses

You may be able to carry out one key statistical analysis that will answer your main research question, and as this is a single analysis, any conclusion will be uncontaminated by multiplicity; that forms a "Primary" analysis. However, during the investigation, you may have collected other data that you would like to consider. Any further statistical tests carried out on the additional data could be acknowledged as being "Secondary" or "Exploratory." You would then be free to carry out as many of these exploratory analyses as you wished, but you would have to emphasize that any apparently statistically significant findings are at increased risk of being false positives and cannot be unduly relied upon. If any positive findings appear to be of practical importance, a further project may be needed to determine whether the original (weak) finding can be confirmed and put on a more secure footing. Often you would describe this as a "need for further work" when discussing these results.

Unscrupulous researchers have been known to work through their list of factors or outcomes and retrospectively select the one that throws up a statistically significant result as their primary outcome. To avoid any accusations of this nature, any distinction between primary and exploratory analyses needs to have been decided upon before the data is seen, and there should be documentary proof that this was the case. It is in this type of situation that pre-registration of experimental plans, such as with a clinical trials registry, or through publication of a study protocol, becomes clearly valuable.

5.2.3 Bonferroni Correction

Sometimes, there may be a good case for using a number of analyses, all of equal status. For example, you might be interested in the possible relationship between social circumstances (measured by employment, household income, cohabitation, and receipt of benefits) and the likelihood of drug misuse. You might judge that no one aspect stood out as an obvious candidate for primary analysis. In such a case, the Bonferroni correction could be applied. This raises the standard of proof, so that any single analysis brings less than a 5% risk of a false positive, and the collection of tests will jointly generate the normal (and acceptable) 5% risk.

The correction is achieved by reducing the critical P-value below the usual 0.05. If the number of tests to be carried out is represented as n, then the corrected critical value (for P) is calculated as:

Corrected critical value = 0.05 / n

So, for example, if you are performing four tests as above, the critical value for P becomes $0.05/4 = 0.0125$. One of the tests might then produce a P-value of (say) 0.03. If this were an isolated test it could be taken to be statistically significant, but as part of a set of four tests, its P-value is greater than 0.0125 and so it should not be considered statistically significant.

6

Common Issues and Pitfalls

6.1 Determining Equality of Standard Deviations

One requirement for procedures such as t-tests and ANOVAs is approximate equality of standard deviations in each of your samples. Moderate differences in SD are tolerable, but if (say) one SD is twice as great as another, then caution is probably wise. If you are seriously concerned that your SDs do differ, there are variant forms of the classical t-test and ANOVA that do not require equal variability.

We do not recommend using formal tests for inequalities among SDs as these are particularly sensitive to sample size and can easily be misinterpreted.

6.2 How Do I Know, in Advance, How Large My SD Will Be?

When calculating necessary sample sizes for work where the outcome will consist of continuously varying data, it is necessary to provide a value for the SD of your samples. How do you know this before actually doing the work? There is no one-size-fits-all solution, but possible routes include:

- Check the literature for work where the same outcome has been recorded, to see how much variability others have encountered. If possible, try to find work carried out under circumstances reasonably similar to those you will use (similar population and sampling strategy).

A Practical Approach to Using Statistics in Health Research: From Planning to Reporting, First Edition. Adam Mackridge and Philip Rowe.
© 2018 John Wiley & Sons, Inc. Published 2018 by John Wiley & Sons, Inc.
Companion website: www.wiley.com/go/Mackridge/
APracticalApproachtoUsingStatisticsinHealthResearch

- Carry out a pilot study to estimate the SD.
- Make an initial, educated guess at the SD, and monitor your data as it comes in to review whether a revision in sample size may be required.

6.3 One-Sided Versus Two-Sided Testing

When investigating a possible difference in a mean value between two groups (A and B), you could simply hypothesize that there will be a difference in the mean, or you could be more specific and say that you think that the mean for A will be bigger than that for B. The first of these scenarios would involve a two-sided question and the second is one-sided. Table 6.1 summarizes one and two-sided testing that could be applied to your data.

Most experienced researchers have met situations where the initial intention was to carry out a two-sided test, but alas, when the data became available, the P-value was somewhere between 0.05 and 0.1. It was then put to them that changing to a one-sided test would halve the P-value and make it "significant." As with any study where the primary analysis is not pre-declared, it is possible to use this approach to return statistically significant findings that are of dubious robustness – see Table 6.1.

Even if you carry out a perfectly fair one-sided test with genuine predetermination of the direction of testing, given the frequent misuse of this approach, you would likely only convince journal referees and anybody who reads your report if you have some written predeclaration of the intention to use a one-sided testing approach.

We would suggest two things:

- For your own work, stick to simple two-sided testing; the gains from one-sided testing aren't worth the bother.
- If you read somebody else's work where they have used a one-sided test and the resulting P-value was significant, but greater than 0.025, then consider this: if they had applied a two-sided test to their data, the P-value would have been greater than 0.05 and therefore nonsignificant. Is there clear evidence that they pre-planned the use of a one-sided test?

For a fuller description of one-sided testing, see Rowe 2015, Chapter 11.[1]

---

[1] Rowe P. Essential statistics for the pharmaceutical sciences, 2nd edn. Chichester: Wiley, 2015.

Table 6.1 Characteristics of one and two-sided questions and testing procedures.

	One-sided (or one-tailed)	Two-sided (or two-tailed)
Question to answer	Either: Is the mean for group A **greater** than that for B? or Is the mean for group A **lower** than that for B?	Is there a difference between the means for groups A and B?
Conditions for a significant conclusion	Any difference must be in the direction suggested by the question **and** Any difference must be sufficiently large.	Any difference must be sufficiently large.
Do you need to declare the direction of difference to be tested for, in advance of seeing the data?	Yes. If any change is then found to be in the opposite direction, the result cannot be claimed as statistically significant.	No.
Is cheating possible?	Yes. Declare the direction of testing *after seeing the data* and choose whatever direction the data suggests. This can convert marginally non-significant data to marginal significance. It also raises the risk of a false positive from the usual 5% to 10%. Do not do it!	No.

6.4 Pitfalls That Make Data Look More Meaningful Than It Really Is

There are a number of ways in which data can be presented that, while not downright dishonest, are none-the-less misleading.

6.4.1 Too Many Decimal Places

Wherever possible, any value for a mean or a percentage should be accompanied by a 95% confidence interval. One good reason (among many others) why this is good practice is that it will remind you that the figure you have just calculated is only an estimate and is subject to random sampling error. You will be a lot less likely to report that "The mean reduction in serum cholesterol levels was 0.78694 mmol/L..." if the next part of that sentence is "(95% confidence interval 0.762 to 0.812 mmol/L.)." Clearly some of those decimal places carry no real information.

All of the following discussion will be couched in terms of "significant digits" and not "decimal places." Table 6.2 presents some examples of rounding to a set number of significant digits.

Most results should be quoted with two or three significant digits. There are two things to bear in mind when deciding how many significant digits to deploy.

- Sampling precision: In the real world, sample estimates are rarely sufficiently precise to justify anything beyond two or three significant digits. A third digit should not be used if the 95% confidence interval suggests that it goes far beyond the precision of your sample value. Thus a value of 12.12 (Confidence interval 7.12 to 17.12) should be rounded to 12; there is huge uncertainty concerning the value and any decimal places would be completely meaningless.
- The use of three significant digits is most likely to be justified with numbers where the first digit is 1, 2, or 3; for numbers beginning

Table 6.2 Rounding to three significant digits.

Initially calculated value	Rounded to three significant digits	Comment
345.123	345	
34.5123	34.5	
0.0034512	0.00345	Leading zeros (Those before the first non-zero digit) are **not** counted as significant digits
345 123	345 000	Trailing zeros are not counted as significant digits
0.120123	0.120	The final zero is significant as it is known to be the best estimate for that digit

with 4 (or anything greater), two significant digits are probably sufficient. This is because the proportional difference between 12 and 12.1 is relatively large and the distinction may be worth making, while for 78 and 78.1, the proportional difference is much smaller and the distinction between the two is unlikely to be practically important.

• Practical usefulness: With very large, precise samples, a fourth or fifth significant digit might be statistically justifiable, but it would be unlikely to serve any useful purpose.

One case where there is justification for the use of three significant digits (or larger numbers) is with percentages greater than 99%. Reporting that a bacterial infection could be cured in 99.7% of patients is not necessarily overly precise; three digits may be required in order to convey the fact that 0.3% cannot be cured.

6.4.2 Percentages with Small Sample Sizes

Statements such as "Three out of four (75%) died." are virtually meaningless: a fact that would be readily appreciated were we to accompany that proportion with its 95% confidence interval (19.4 to 99.4%). In other words, the true proportion could be almost anything! You should not quote percentages based on very small samples. If ten out of twenty patients died, then even with this sample size, the 95% confidence interval for the case fatality rate is 27.2 to 72.8%; the estimate is still very imprecise. A sample size of 20 would be the absolute minimum for the calculation of a meaningful percentage.

Percentages should certainly not be quoted with decimal places where the sample size was less than 100.

6.5 Discussion of Statistically Significant Results

The word "Significant" is dangerously ambiguous. In the context of statistical significance, it is merely evidence that there is a relationship between an outcome and a factor. It gives no indication as to whether this is of any practical or clinical relevance. To judge practical relevance, it is essential to have a measure of effect size and its confidence interval. This measure of effect size should then be used to determine whether the change in outcome is large enough to be of practical relevance.

- In the case of a continuously varying measured outcome, the measure of effect size would probably be the difference between the mean values for two study groups.
- For a categorical outcome, it could be the Relative Risk, Odds Ratio or Number Needed to Treat (See Section 7.9).
- Ways to describe ordinal data are discussed in Section 3.2. One approach would be to use the proportion above/below some crucial point on the ordinal scale. The outcomes then become simple categorizations (above/below the crucial value) and the Relative Risk or Odds Ratio etc. can be used to express the effect size.

Figure 6.1 shows some hypothetical differences in outcome comparing active versus control treatment where the endpoint is diastolic blood pressure (a continuously varying measure). It is assumed that the smallest difference that would be of practically relevance (often termed the Clinically Relevant Difference – CRD) is 5 mmHg. These limits are indicated by the vertical broken lines; any change between these limits can be considered trivial, and interventions achieving such small changes would not be likely to be adopted into practice.

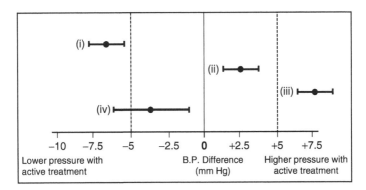

Figure 6.1 Hypothetical confidence intervals for the difference in blood pressure between actively treated and control patients. All are statistically significant (the null hypothesis figure of zero is excluded from the confidence interval), but their interpretations differ. Vertical broken lines indicate limits beyond which differences would be of practical/clinical significance.

Example (i) Shows a practically relevant reduction in blood pressure; even the smallest effect suggested by the confidence interval (approximately -6 mmHg) is large enough to be of practical relevance. Case (iii) shows a relevant increase in blood pressure. With (ii) we have statistical significance (the confidence interval does not cross the zero-difference line), but the effect is trivially small – not of practical relevance. Case (iv) is less clear cut; the probability is that the effect is trivial, but there is some remaining possibility that the reduction in blood pressure could be great enough to be practically relevant.

In your discussion, you should not simply say the result was "significant" as this may be read as implying practical significance when this may not be the case. It is far better to describe this as "statistically significant" and ensure that the practical or clinical relevance is discussed alongside this.

Figure 6.2 is similar to Figure 6.1, but considers a categorical outcome such as death. The effect size has been expressed as the Relative Risk (RR). Here it is assumed that changes to the RR are only of practical relevance if the risk is at least halved or doubled. Cases (i) and (iii) show a reduction and increase respectively in risk, each of which is large enough to be of practical consequence. With case (ii) there is a change in risk, but it is not practically relevant. For case (iv) the change in risk is probably of real consequence, but some doubt remains.

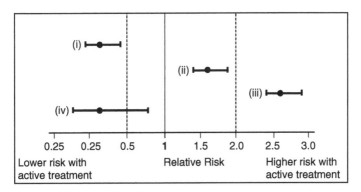

Figure 6.2 Hypothetical confidence intervals for the relative risk of death for actively treated patients compared to controls. All are statistically significant (the null hypothesis figure of one is excluded from the confidence interval), but their interpretations differ. Vertical broken lines indicate limits beyond which differences would be of practical/clinical significance.

6.6 Discussion of Non-Significant Results

Statistical non-significance does not necessarily mean that there is no change in outcome between the different factors; it means that your data did not *show* a change. Failure to show a change may arise because there was none or because you failed to detect it – typically because the sample size was too small. As in the previous section, the only way to interpret the result is by inspection of the confidence interval for the effect size, also bearing in mind the practically/clinically relevant difference.

Figure 6.3 is structured in a similar manner to Figure 6.1, but these cases are all statistically non-significant. For case (i), the result is not merely statistically non-significant; we can say with confidence that there is no effect of any real consequence. Case (ii) shows a very wide confidence interval. This only narrowly misses statistical significance, and there is a considerable possibility of a change that is big enough to be of practical consequence. Further work with larger sample sizes would be justified. With case (iii), if there is any effect at all, it is proba-bly trivially small, with only a slight residual possibility of a meaningful difference; further work would be unlikely to reveal any worthwhile effect.

Figure 6.4 shows statistically non-significant outcomes for a cate-gorical outcome. Case (i) excludes the possibility of any practically

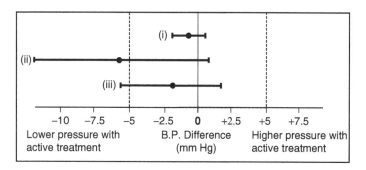

Figure 6.3 Hypothetical confidence intervals for the difference in blood pressure between actively treated and control patients. All are statistically non-significant (the null hypothesis figure of zero is included by the confidence interval), but their interpretations differ. Vertical broken lines indicate limits beyond which differences would be of practical/clinical significance.

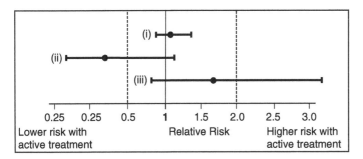

Figure 6.4 Hypothetical confidence intervals for the relative risk of death for actively treated patients compared to controls. All are statistically non-significant significant (the null hypothesis figure of one is included by the confidence interval), but their interpretations differ. Vertical broken lines indicate limits beyond which differences would be of practical/clinical significance.

relevant change in risk. Case (ii) leaves a considerable chance that there might be an effect that achieves practical significance, and (iii) shows a wide confidence interval, which leaves a worrying possibility that the active treatment might be causing some real harm. With both cases (ii) and (iii), further work with larger sample sizes would be useful.

6.7 Describing Effect Sizes with Non-Parametric Tests

Non-parametric methods generally do not generate any useful confidence interval for the effect size, so you will probably not be able to follow fully the recommendations in Sections 6.5 and 6.6. Some suggestions follow.

- For a non-significant result: If sample sizes are small, be wary of saying there is no effect; one may be present but you have failed to detect it. With large samples, you can more safely say that there is either no effect or, at the very least, any effect is very small and therefore probably not of any practical relevance.
- For a significant result: Discuss whether the effect size is great enough to be of practical consequence and its implications for public policy or professional practice.

Rowe (2015, Section 21.2.5) discusses in detail the interpretation of a statistically significant finding with a non-parametric test. It is always safe to use wording such as "Values for the endpoint are higher in group A than in group B." However, any claim that the median or mean is higher in one group than in the other would only be reliable if the distributions of the two sets of data were appropriate, so caution is needed.

6.8 Confusing Association with a Cause and Effect Relationship

If your experimental design involves randomizing individuals or institutions to different treatment groups, you can be fairly sure that your two (or more) study groups will differ only in regards to the treatment received. If you then find significant evidence of a difference between groups, it should be safe to conclude that there is a cause and effect relationship between the treatment and the outcome.

Where allocation is not random and/or other sources of bias have not been adequately controlled in the study design, it is possible that the study groups differ in ways other than the specific characteristic that the study is intended to address. There is therefore always some danger attached to any claim that a demonstrated difference between the groups was caused by the specific factor that you used to distinguish the two groups. As such, it is reasonable to describe an *association* or *relationship* between the factor and outcome, but it is not possible to say with confidence that this is *causative*.

An example of this would be the relationship between the day of admission to hospital and the likelihood that a patient will die during their hospital stay – in studies of this, there is a statistically and practically significant increased risk of death among patients admitted at the weekend. However, there is a strong possibility of bias in the allocation of patients to "admission on a weekday" vs. "admission at a weekend" – for example, people admitted outside of normal service hours may be more likely to be suffering from severe illness, which may be the primary factor leading to their increased death rates. As such, unless this and other important sources of bias have been controlled for, it would not be appropriate to say that the increase in death rate is attributable to the day of admission.

Where there is a credible mechanism by which the alleged causal factor could bring about the observed difference in outcomes, this may strengthen the case considerably, but caution is still needed.

Correlations (Chapters 18–20) are particularly liable to turn out to be mere associations and not true cause/effect relationships as randomization is rarely a feature.

7

Contingency Chi-Square Test

7.1 When Is the Test Appropriate?

Figure 7.1 shows the circumstances where a chi-square test is used:

- The factor is categorical; the figure shows two groups, and these might be categories such as Treated/Untreated, Exposed/Unexposed, Male/Female etc. The chi-square test will allow you to analyze three or more groups, but interpretation is easiest with two.
- The outcome is categorical; the figure again shows just two possibilities (A and B), which might be something like Survived/Died, Satisfied/Unsatisfied, Success/Failure etc. Again, there could be more, but interpretation is easiest with just two.
- Each participant provides just one outcome result – Participants A…H under condition 1 and I…O under condition 2 (data sets are independent/unpaired).
- What is being tested is the apparently greater occurrence of outcome A under condition 1 than under condition 2.

Some examples are shown in Table 7.1. For full details of the test see Rowe (2015) Chapter 18, Sections 1 to 5.

7.2 An Example

Elderly patients undergoing cardiac surgery were randomized to receive either normal care or normal care plus a package of physiotherapy and

A Practical Approach to Using Statistics in Health Research: From Planning to Reporting, First Edition. Adam Mackridge and Philip Rowe.
© 2018 John Wiley & Sons, Inc. Published 2018 by John Wiley & Sons, Inc.
Companion website: www.wiley.com/go/Mackridge/
APracticalApproachtoUsingStatisticsinHealthResearch

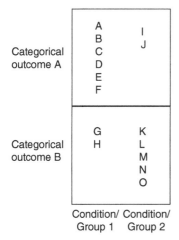

Figure 7.1 Experimental structure where a contingency chi-square test is appropriate.

Table 7.1 Examples of studies that would be analyzed by a contingency chi-square test.

Groups compared	Outcome	Question
Patients using new form of walking aid versus those using current standard equipment	Do or do not experience a fall during hospital stay	Does the choice of walking aid influence the risk of falls?
Nicotine users from most deprived quintile versus those from least deprived quintile	Smoke tobacco or use e-cigarettes	Is use of e-cigarettes among nicotine users associated with level of deprivation?
GP practices employing a practice pharmacist versus those that do not employ a practice pharmacist	Target for patient access to appointments is met or not met	Is patient access to appointments in GP practices linked to employment of a practice pharmacist?
Patients trained by doctors or nurses to use an inhaler	Satisfactory or unsatisfactory technique for inhaler use	Are those trained by one professional group more successful than those trained by the other?

exercise to improve fitness before their surgery. The recorded outcome was whether the patient did or did not develop post-operative pneumonia within the follow up period. The data are available as an MS Excel spreadsheet or SPSS data file; See last section of this chapter.

7.3 Presenting the Data

The data could be presented in a tabular or visual form – See Table 7.2 and Figure 7.2 and 7.3. With our example data, either approach illustrates a lower proportion experiencing pneumonia among those receiving the physiotherapy and exercise intervention.

7.3.1 Contingency Tables

In Table 7.2, the results of the example study are shown as a contingency table. It is vital that the actual count for each cell is included. It is also very useful to include the percentages for the various outcomes in each group.

7.3.2 Clustered or Stacked Bar Charts

Figures 7.2 and 7.3 show clustered and stacked bar charts of the current data. Notice that while Figure 7.2 does provide the actual counts, Figure 7.3 only presents the proportions, not the counts; it would be vital to accompany the latter figure with a statement of the sample sizes for the two groups under comparison.

Table 7.2 Contingency table showing numbers and percentages with and without pneumonia among patients who do or do not receive physiotherapy and exercise in addition to normal care.

	Usual care only	Additional physiotherapy and exercise
Without pneumonia	190 (83.0%)	199 (91.7%)
With pneumonia	39 (17.0%)	18 (8.3%)

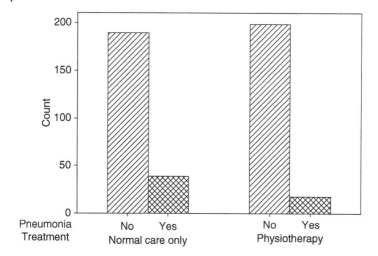

Figure 7.2 Clustered bar chart showing numbers with and without pneumonia among cardiac surgery patients who do or do not receive physiotherapy and exercise in addition to normal care.

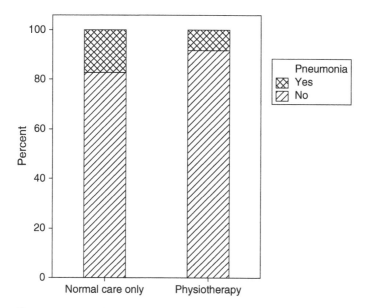

Figure 7.3 Stacked bar chart showing proportions with and without pneumonia among cardiac surgery patients who do or do not receive physiotherapy and exercise in addition to normal care.

7.4   Data Requirements

You will use two categorical variables, one recording group membership and the other recording the outcome. Normal distributions are not relevant for categorical data, so there are no requirements in this respect.

7.5   An Outline of the Test

Three aspects of the data will determine whether your results are statistically significant:

- The extent of the contrast between the proportions in the two groups. Large differences are more likely to be judged significant than small ones.
- The size of your samples. Large samples are more likely to return significant results than small ones.
- Is one of the outcomes always rare? If only a very small proportion of patients in both groups developed pneumonia, you would observe only small numbers of positive cases, and your estimates of the proportions in this category would be imprecise. The result is therefore less likely to be returned as significant. Significance is most easily achieved if all categories are reasonably common.

7.6   Planning Sample Sizes

To calculate necessary sample sizes, you will need to provide four values:

- The baseline proportion of individuals that you expect to fall into one of the categories in one of your study groups. In the present example, you could provide the proportion you anticipate will suffer pneumonia in the control group (those receiving usual care). Let us say that you anticipate a 25% rate of pneumonia in the control group.
- The smallest difference between the two groups that you wish to be able to detect. You would indicate this as a proportion in the other group. If you quoted a figure of 12.5% for the intervention group, you would power your trial to allow the detection of a reduction of the rate of pneumonia from 25% in the controls to 12.5% or less in the intervention group.

- The power you require. The more power you request, the larger your sample sizes will need to be. This is usually within the range 80-95%, but using 90% is normally a good choice, unless you have special reasons to select anything else.
- What P-value[1] you will consider as statistically significant. Typically, a P-value of less than 0.05 is appropriate.

The figures quoted above generate a necessary sample size of 216. This is the number in each experimental group, so at least 432 participants are required to complete the study. You may need to increase this figure further as a recruitment target to allow for participant drop outs between recruitment and completion of the study. The degree to which this is necessary would depend on how likely it is that participants would drop out from your study – for a questionnaire survey, dropout from agreement to completion is generally low, but for a clinical intervention study, over a number of months, drop out could be quite large (30% or more). You can use known drop out figures from existing studies, where available, or estimate this based on experience or other studies with similar requirements on the participants.

See video listed at end of chapter for detailed instructions on calculating sample sizes.

7.7 Carrying Out the Test

For most packages (including SPSS), the data is entered in two columns: one recording the group to which a participant/institution belongs (in the current case, Normal treatment only or Additional intervention) and another column for that participant's outcome (currently, With or Without pneumonia). Alternatively, if you already have the data as a contingency table, the cell counts can be entered in the same pattern as in Table 7.2. The latter is referred to as "summarized" format.

The outcome of the test is P = 0.009, which is statistically significant.

See the video listed at end of chapter for detailed instructions on carrying out the chi-square test.

---

[1] The p-value may be referred to in software packages as "Alpha" – See glossary.

7.8   Special Issues

7.8.1   Yates Correction

The mathematical calculations within the chi-square test assume that the observed numbers of individuals are continuous (e.g. we could observe 13.75 patients with pneumonia). The reality is that we can actually only observe whole numbers. This slightly biases the test in favor of a significant outcome. The Yates correction compensates for this by reducing the likelihood of significance. However, the correction can be too powerful and may make the test return a false negative. We recommend applying Yates' correction only to contingency tables with two columns and two rows. For larger tables (three or more rows or three or more columns), do not apply it.

In the video mentioned above, you will be shown how to obtain the Yates-corrected results.

7.8.2   Low Expected Frequencies – Fisher's Exact Test

When the software calculates the chi-square test, it generates something called "Expected frequencies" (see glossary) and, if any of these are below five, the chi-square test result can be unreliable. Note that it is the expected frequencies you need to consider; it does not necessarily matter if some of the actual observed frequencies in your contingency table are less than five. Most statistical packages will issue a warning if any expected frequencies are below five.

Fortunately, there is an alternative test – Fisher's exact test – that will answer the same research question, and it does not involve the calculation of expected frequencies, so this problem is avoided. In the video, you will be shown how to determine whether a switch to Fisher's exact test is required and how to obtain the results of the alternative test.

7.9   Describing the Effect Size

In the discussion that follows, there will be reference to the "Event." You will have to decide, for your study, which outcome is the "Event" and which the "Non-event." For our study, we will treat pneumonia as the event, but we could have chosen avoidance of pneumonia as the event.

There are several ways to describe effect sizes when the outcome is categorical. You need to consider which is most effective with your data set. Part of your consideration should be whether, in your area of study, it is custom and practice to use one particular method; it would be helpful to make your results as comparable as possible with the existing literature. If you are uncertain which method to use, most of your readers will find it easy to comprehend the Relative Risk (RR).

In the following sections, note the technical use of the word "Risk"; it is simply used to mean the likelihood of the event. This is fine when the event is something undesirable such as death or disease. However, the same word is also commonly used for the likelihood of desirable outcomes such as affecting a cure or conceiving a child when this was intended. You need to get used to the idea of the "Risk of being cured" – it simply refers to its likelihood.

The various different ways to describe effect size are summarized below, but you should see Rowe (2015; Chapter 19)[1] for full details of the various methods. The video listed at the end of this chapter shows how to obtain these measures of effect size and their 95% confidence intervals.

> If your study is of the case:control type, you must see section 7.9.5.

7.9.1   Absolute Risk Difference (ARD)

This is simply:

(Proportion with the event in the intervention/exposed group) – (Proportion with the event in the control/unexposed group).

Note the convention that it is Intervention minus Control. The ARD can be expressed as either a proportion or a percentage. If you express it as a percentage, be careful with your wording. If the percentage with the event fell from 60% to 30%, you should not report this as "There was a reduction of 30%" as this may be misunderstood as meaning a reduction in the risk of the event by just under one third, when the risk actually falls by half. It would be much less ambiguous to say "There was an absolute reduction of 30 percentage points."

---

[1]   Rowe P. Essential statistics for the pharmaceutical sciences, 2nd edn. Chichester: Wiley, 2015.

In the current example, pre-operative physiotherapy and exercise were associated with a reduction in the rate of pneumonia from 17.0% to 8.3%, giving an ARD of -8.7 percentage points. ARD is sometimes also shown as a decimal fraction – in this case, -0.087.

The 95% confidence interval for the effect of additional treatment is a change in the incidence of pneumonia by anything between -2.6 and -14.8 percentage points. The confidence interval can be calculated using a spreadsheet, which is available on our companion website – see the end of this chapter for details on how to access this.

7.9.2   Number Needed to Treat (NNT)

This is the number of patients we would need to switch from one set of circumstances to another in order to achieve one additional favorable outcome event (in this case, one more case avoiding pneumonia). It is calculated as:

1 / ARD

Any fractional value is always rounded upwards to a whole number. For the current study:

NNT = 1 / 0.087 = 11.5

Thus the NNT is rounded to twelve and we would need to provide the intervention to twelve additional patients in order to avoid one case of pneumonia.

Confidence intervals for NNTs are best avoided as they may be excessively sensitive to changes in the categorization of a single individual, which can dramatically change the confidence limits.

7.9.3   Risk Ratio (RR)

This is also known as the "Relative Risk" or "Rate Ratio." It is calculated as:

(Proportion with the event in the intervention/exposed group) / (Proportion with the event in the control/unexposed group).

Note the convention of using Intervention divided by Control. For the current study:

RR = 17.0% / 8.3% = 0.49

A Risk Ratio of 0.49 tells the reader that the intervention caused an approximate halving in the likelihood of pneumonia.

The 95% CI for the RR is 0.29 to 0.83. This is obtainable from SPSS via the instructions given in the videos at the end of the chapter.

It can be misleading to quote the RR in cases where the risk is low. For example, if a normal, law-abiding member of the British public wore a bullet proof jacket at all times, the risk of being fatally shot during a twelve month period might be reduced from one in ten million to one in fifty million. Quoting an RR of 0.2 makes it sound like a wise precaution, but the NNT (12.5 million) conveys its sheer futility.

7.9.4 Odds Ratio (OR)

First calculate the odds for each group as:

$$Odds = \frac{(Proportion\ with\ the\ event)}{(Proportion\ without\ the\ event)}$$

Then calculate the odds ratio as:

$$\frac{(Odds\ for\ the\ intervention\,/\,exposed\ group)}{(Odds\ for\ the\ control\,/\,unexposed\ group)}$$

In this study:

Odds of pneumonia for the intervention group = 8.3% / 91.7% =.0905
Odds of pneumonia for the comparator group = 17.0% / 83.0% = 0.2048
Odds ratio = 0.0905 / 0.2048 = 0.44

An OR less than one tells the reader that the intervention reduced the likelihood of pneumonia. For many readers, the OR will be less intuitive than the RR, but where the event is uncommon (say, less than 10% in both study groups), the OR and RR are numerically almost equal and the OR can be interpreted virtually as if it was the RR (see Rowe 2015 Section 19.2).

The 95% CI for the OR is 0.24 to 0.80. This is obtainable from SPSS using the instructions given in the videos listed at the end of the chapter.

The null hypothesis (where the intervention has no effect) figure for both the RR and the OR is 1.0.

7.9.5 Case: Control Studies

Case: control studies are generally used in epidemiology. Two sets of subjects are selected, with one group containing individuals who have undergone a specified event – usually the development of a clinical condition – and those in the other group having not undergone the relevant event. The investigator then determines retrospectively whether each individual had been exposed to a particular circumstance that is suspected of changing the risk of the event. The question is then whether there is a difference in the proportions of those exposed and non-exposed in the two outcome groups. In these studies, the samples do not estimate the risk of the event among either the exposed or nonexposed individuals in the general population. It is therefore impossible to calculate the ARD, NNT or RR. However, it is possible to calculate the OR, and this is the indicator of effect size that is generally used.

7.10   How to Report the Analysis

7.10.1   Methods

You should include all of the following:

- How your sample size was calculated. (If it was not pre-calculated, say why not; maybe all available cases in a pre-existing database were used.)
- The variable used to divide the cases (patients or institutions) into groups (factor).
- The variable used to record the outcome.
- The name of the statistical analysis employed (use the exact same wording as that in the menu structure of the package you used).
- Options selected (if any are different from the program's defaults).
- The P-value that would be considered as statistically significant.
- The name of your statistical package along with its version number and supplier.

Suitable wording might be:

> Minimum sample sizes of 216 per group were calculated using the G*Power software (Heinrich-Heine-Universität Düsseldorf), based on assumptions that there would be an approximately 25% incidence of pneumonia in the control group *(give references or justification)* and that a reduction to 12.5% in the intervention group would be clinically meaningful *(references or justification)*. The a priori P-value was set at less than 0.05 and a power of 90% used in the calculation.
>
> The proportions with pneumonia in the two groups were compared using the Crosstabs routine with the addition of a chi-square test (SPSS Version 23; IBM Corporation).

7.10.2   Results

You should include all of the following:

- The sample sizes used.
- The contingency table along with percentages for the various outcomes in each group and/or a clustered or stacked bar chart.
- If Fisher's exact test was used, describe the low expected frequencies that lead to its use and report the P-value.
- If the chi-square test was used, the value of the test-statistic (chi-square) may be reported but it can be left out in most cases; however, you must report the P-value.
- Where a chi-square test was used, whether Yates' correction was applied.
- A statement as to whether statistical significance was achieved.
- An appropriate measure of effect size such as the ARD, RR, OR or NNT (or a combination of these). A 95% confidence interval should be included (unless the NNT is being used).

Suitable wording might be:

> The numbers of valid participants and proportions suffering pneumonia in the two patient groups are shown in Table 7.2 *(or Figure 7.2)*. There was a statistically significantly (Yates corrected P-value = 0.009) reduced incidence of pneumonia in the intervention group with the relative risk of pneumonia in the additional physiotherapy group being 0.49 (95% CI 0.29 to 0.83).

7.10.3 Discussion

It would be appropriate to explore the following points relating to your statistical analysis. Within this, you will need to provide and justify a value for the clinically/practically relevant difference.

- See Sections 6.5 and 6.6 for guidance on interpreting statistically significant or non-significant results.
- Whether or not statistically significant – the implications for public policy or professional practice.

7.11 Confounding and Logistic Regression

A commonly quoted example of confounding is the observation that the rate of lung cancer is higher among participants who carry matches than among those who do not, and yet only a fool would conclude that matches cause cancer – it is simply the fact that people who smoke tobacco (the likely cause of increased cancer risk) are much more likely to carry matches than those who do not smoke. The general feature of confounding is that two characteristics are associated with each other, but there is no direct causal relationship. Typically, this is because they share a third characteristic, which is the true causative factor – finding this can often be the hardest part of epidemiological or observational research where participants are not randomized to a particular group. In these studies, the investigator has no control over the group to which each participant belongs. It is then perfectly possible (in fact vey common) for the study groups to differ in several characteristics in addition to the one you are trying to study.

If you carry out an observational/epidemiological study and perform a series of chi-square tests, you may identify several factors as having statistically significant relationships with a particular outcome. However, you would have to consider the possibility that some of these factors might be confounded with each other. In such a case, you should combine those factors into a single logistic regression analysis. This is a technique that can consider several alleged factors within a single analysis and distinguish between those factors that are merely confounded and those that are directly related to the outcome. For example, if you included both match carrying and smoking status as possible factors and lung cancer as the outcome, this should confirm smoking as directly associated with the cancer, but reject match carrying. Logistic regression would take account of the fact that individuals who smoked but did not carry matches had just as high a risk of cancer as those who smoked and did carry matches, and so the matches had nothing to do with the cancer.

If a combined logistic regression dismisses one of the factors as non-significant, it should not be claimed as having a causal relationship with the outcome, even if it was apparently significant when analyzed in isolation in a chi-square test.

For a more comprehensive explanation (especially of logistic regression), see our sister publication (Rowe 2015) section 20.2. A video listed at the end of this chapter gives details of executing a logistic regression.

7.11.1 Reporting the Detection of Confounding

In the methods section, you need to describe each of the following unless they have already been reported elsewhere in your report:

- The outcome that was observed.
- The various factors that were tested.
- The name of the statistical analysis employed (use the exact same wording as that in the menu structure of the package you used).
- The name of your statistical package along with its version number and supplier.
- The P-value that would be considered statistically significant.

Suitable additional wording in the methods section might be:

> Binary logistic regression was performed using SPSS (Version 23; IBM Corporation) with lung cancer as the outcome and the carrying of matches and smoking as factors. An a priori value of P <0.05 was considered statistically significant.

In the results section you need to report the P-values for each of the possible factors and offer a diagnosis as to whether each had a genuinely independent effect or was confounded. Suitable wording might be:

> Results: Binary logistic regression considering both factors simultaneously identified smoking as having a direct relationship with lung cancer (P = 0.001) but that there was no direct relationship between lung cancer and match-carrying (P = 0.71).

7.12   Larger Tables

Table 7.2 has just two rows (Without or With pneumonia) and two columns (With pre-operative physiotherapy and exercise or Usual care). This is referred to as "Two-by-two" (or 2x2) and is the smallest possible contingency table, but it is possible to have one or more additional column(s) or row(s), making a three-way (or more) comparison. For example, we could have a table with three study groups ("Normal care," two different packages of pre-operative physiotherapy & exercise), and three outcomes of "No pneumonia," "Pneumonia (successfully treated)" and "Pneumonia (fatal)".

The chi-square test can be applied to these larger tables, but the Yates correction is not applicable (See section 7.8.1). However, there is a big difference in the ease of interpretation of the outcome. If you obtain a statistically significant result for a 2x2 table such as Table 7.2, the only possible interpretation is that pre-operative physiotherapy & exercise reduces the risk of pneumonia. However, if you increased both the number of rows and columns to three (as suggested in the previous paragraph), a significant result would be less easily interpreted. Is the real difference between the comparator and intervention 1, between the comparator and intervention 2, or between the two intervention methods? Similarly, is the significant difference between the rates of no pneumonia and non-fatal pneumonia or some other contrast?

There is a further problem; with larger tables, you cannot calculate measures of effect size such as the risk ratio or odds ratio in the simple and unambiguous way that was shown in section 7.9.

Given these issues, it is wise to try to design your study to generate 2x2 tables, such that your findings are clearly interpretable and more likely to be useful to practice or policy.

7.12.1   Collapsing Tables

It can be quite tempting to indulge in "collapsing" large contingency tables. For instance, if we had created three outcomes of No pneumonia, Treatable pneumonia and Fatal pneumonia, we could reduce the size and complexity of the table by combining the last two categories, leaving us with just With/Without pneumonia. However, we might also decide to collapse the table to Survived/Died. This introduces possible multiple testing and increased risk of false positives as outlined in Chapter 5. With very complex tables that do not achieve statistical significance, there is a good chance of hitting upon some form of collapsing that does give apparent significance. Collapsing of tables should be used judiciously and, unless pre-planned, reported appropriately as a secondary analysis.

It has to be recognized that investigators using pre-existing databases may well be faced with data structures of considerable complexity, where collapsing of categories is an essential step toward making any sense of the results. A few points to consider follow:

- Ideally, the specific form of collapsing would have been pre-planned before the results were seen.
- If the full table is already statistically significant and the goal is simply to identify where significance lies or allow the calculation of an effect size such as relative risk, there should be no great objection.
- If the data structure allows few logical patterns of collapsing, the problem is less serious.
- If none of the above apply, but collapsing of categories is judged essential, then the risk of false positive findings must be addressed within the discussion and any statistically significant findings treated with due modesty.

7 12.2   Reducing Tables

Let us say that you performed the physiotherapy trial with three treatments (Control, Physiotherapy package 1 and Physiotherapy package 2) and outcomes of Pneumonia /No pneumonia, and you achieved statistical significance. All you would know was that there was at least one treatment that differed from one other, but which of the possible comparisons (Control v Treatment 1; Control v Treatment 2; Treatment 1 v Treatment 2) were significant? It could be any one (or several) of these.

One approach would be to reduce the 2x3 table to a 2x2 table by omitting Treatment 2. You could then use another chi-square test to unambiguously compare control versus Treatment 1. Similar maneuvers could then be used to compare Control versus Treatment 2 and Treatment 1 versus Treatment 2 (a total of three tests). However, this now constitutes multiple testing, and you would need to apply the

Bonferroni correction (Section 5.2.3), only claiming statistical significance if P < 0.0167. While this approach is technically valid, we would still recommend sticking to simple, easily interpreted studies that will fit into a 2x2 table.

7.13   Relevant Videos etc.

The following are available at
www.wiley.com/go/Mackridge/APracticalApproachtoUsingStatisticsin
HealthResearch

Videos

Video_1.1_SPSS_Basics: The absolute basics of using SPSS

Video_7.1_ChiSquare_SampSize: Using G*Power for chi-square sample size calculation

Video_7.2_ChiSquareTest: Using SPSS for contingency tables, chi-square test, Yates correction, Fisher's exact test, and Relative Risk etc. plus confidence intervals

Video_7.3_DetectingConfounding: Using SPSS for logistic regression to detect confounding

SPSS data files

SPSS_7.1_PhysiotherapyPneumonia: The data for the example used to illustrate this chapter

Spreadsheets

Spreadsheet_7.1_PhysiotherapyPneumonia.xlsx: The data for the example used to illustrate this chapter

Spreadsheet_7.2_RR_OR_NNT_Calculator.xlsx. Spreadsheet for calculating Relative Risk, Odds Ratio, and Number Needed to Treat and 95% confidence intervals

8

Independent Samples (Two-Sample) T-Test

The terms "Independent samples t-test" and "Two-sample t-test" are entirely interchangeable, describing the same test.

8.1   When Is the Test Applied?

Figure 8.1 shows the circumstances where a two-sample t-test is used:

- There are **two** categorically different conditions or groups (factor).
- The outcome is a continuously varying measure.
- Each subject provides just one outcome result – Subjects A…E under condition 1 and F…J under condition 2.
- What is being tested is the appearance that there are greater values for the measured outcome under one condition than under the other.

Some examples where this test is appropriate are shown in Table 8.1

8.2   An Example

In our example, we take the last case in Table 8.1. We have used a visual analog scale to determine the level of pain being experienced by women 24 hours after either abdominal or laparoscopic hysterectomy. The scale produces scores of between 0 and 100, where 100 represents the highest level of pain. (The dataset is available as an MS Excel spreadsheet and an SPSS data file listed at the end of this chapter.)

A Practical Approach to Using Statistics in Health Research: From Planning to Reporting, First Edition. Adam Mackridge and Philip Rowe.
© 2018 John Wiley & Sons, Inc. Published 2018 by John Wiley & Sons, Inc.
Companion website: www.wiley.com/go/Mackridge/
APracticalApproachtoUsingStatisticsinHealthResearch

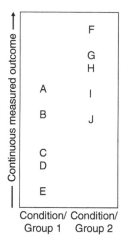

Figure 8.1 Circumstances when an independent samples t-test is used.

Table 8.1 Examples of studies that would be analyzed by an independent samples (two-sample) t-test.

Comparison made	Outcome	Question
People in a group who use a cholesterol lowering spread in place of butter for a three month period versus another group who make no change.	Change in serum cholesterol between beginning and end of study period.	Does the experimental spread influence serum cholesterol levels?
Hospitalized patients receiving routine care versus those receiving additional planned nurse review every one to two hours.	Score on a standardized questionnaire assessing patient satisfaction with nursing care.	Is the additional planned attention reflected in a change in patient satisfaction with nursing care?
Patients with lower back pain given access to an eight-week program of physiotherapy versus those not given such access.	Change in score between beginning and end of study period on a standardized functional disability questionnaire.	Does access to physiotherapy change levels of functional disability in such patients?
Patients undergoing laparoscopic versus those having abdominal hysterectomies.	Visual analog scale for pain 24 hours post-surgery.	Are pain levels different according to mode of surgery?

8.3   Presenting the Data

8.3.1   Numerically

You should report the sample size, mean, and standard deviation for the outcome in both study groups. You should also report the difference between the two sample means and its 95% confidence interval. The final point is vital and might be reported as "The estimated difference between the mean pain levels for the two groups was 14.4 points (95% confidence interval 8.5 to 20.4 points), positive values representing higher pain in the abdominal surgery group."

8.3.2   Graphically

For a general discussion of how to present continuously varying measured data, see Chapter 3. You would probably use histograms or dot plots. Histograms require reasonably large data sets to work effectively. Dot plots may be the only effective way to represent small data sets. In the current case, there is enough data to produce effective histograms (Figure 8.2). These show apparently lower pain levels with the laparoscopic procedure.

8.4   Data Requirements

8.4.1   Variables Required

Almost all statistical software programs will accept the data stored as two variables (columns in SPSS).

- A categorical variable will be used to divide the subjects into two groups: in our case, this describes which surgical procedure was used (Laparoscopic or Abdominal).
- A continuous measured variable to record the outcome: the visual analog pain scores (0–100).

8.4.2   Normal Distribution of the Outcome Variable Within the Two Samples

It is a requirement that each of your samples should be approximately normally distributed. See Chapter two for a general discussion of the

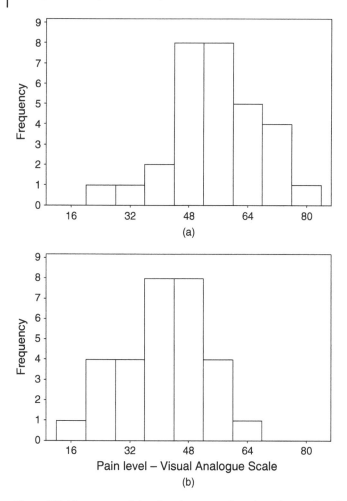

Figure 8.2 Histograms of visual analog scores for pain 24 hours after abdominal or laparoscopic hysterectomy. (a) Abdominal, (b) Laparoscopic.

detection of non-normal distribution using histograms and normal probability plots. The distributions in Figure 8.2 show approximately normal distributions, and normal probability plots of this data (Figure 8.3) show no signs of long-tailed distributions.

Notice that you must check for normality in both data sets separately. If the two study groups are each normally distributed and have

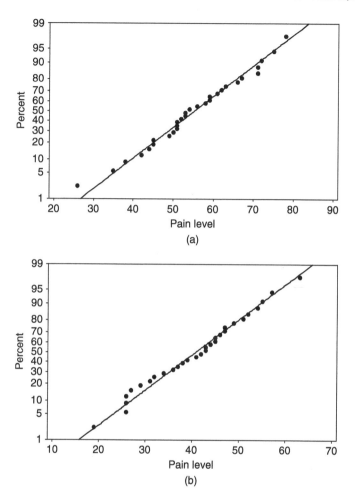

Figure 8.3 Normal probability plots of pain data following (a) Abdominal or (b) Laparoscopic hysterectomy.

different means, then a combination of both data sets will not be normally distributed.

With this example data, there is no evidence of any of the problems mentioned in Chapter 2, and it is reasonable to treat the data as adequately approximating a normal distribution.

If data is severely non-normal due to positive skew, it may be possible to convert the data to normality using the log-transform. A video listed at the end of this chapter gives details of using SPSS to check for normality and for log transformation of non-normal data to normality. If the data cannot be transformed to normality, you should use the non-parametric Mann–Whitney test (see Chapter 9).

8.4.3 Equal Standard Deviations

For a classical t-test, it is also a condition that your samples have approximately equal standard deviations (SDs). See Section 6.1 for a general discussion of detection of unequal SDs. If problems arise, there is an alternative form of the test (Welch's approximate t-test) that is tolerant of differing SDs. However, with approximately similar SDs, it is best to use the classical t-test, as it is a little more powerful. Switching to Welch's test is covered in a video listed at the end of this chapter. With the current data, the SDs for the two samples are acceptably similar (±12.2 and 10.7).

8.4.4 Equal Sample Sizes

Equality of sample sizes is not a condition for the independent samples t-test. However, for any given total number of observations, statistical power is greatest with the data divided equally between the two samples.

8.5 An Outline of the Test

Three aspects of the data will determine whether your results are statistically significant:

- The size of difference between the two sample means: A small difference is likely to be dismissed as statistically non-significant, while a large difference is more likely to achieve significance.
- The size of your samples: It is very difficult for small samples to provide adequate evidence of a real difference, whereas large samples are more likely to result in statistical significance.

- The standard deviation within each sample: Highly varying data (large standard deviation) leaves greater uncertainty as to the true mean value for each group, and hence it is harder to be sure there is a real difference between them.

8.6 Planning Sample Sizes

To calculate necessary sample sizes, you will need to provide four values:

- The smallest difference between the two means that you wish to be able to detect. This will probably be the Clinically Relevant Difference (See glossary). Small differences are hard to detect, and large samples will be needed; large differences stand out clearly, and even small samples will suffice.
- The anticipated standard deviation in the two samples – see Section 6.2.
- The power you require – see glossary. The more power you require, the larger your sample sizes will need to be. For most purposes, 90% power is a reasonable figure.
- The P-value you will consider as statistically significant. Most statistical packages use a default value of 0.05. The program may refer to this as "Alpha" – see glossary.

See a video listed at the end of this chapter for detailed instructions on using G*Power to calculate sample sizes.

8.7 Carrying Out the Test

See a video listed at the end of this chapter for detailed instructions on carrying out the t-test.

8.8 Describing the Effect Size

The effect size is described as the estimated difference between the two group means and its 95% confidence interval. In the hysterectomy example, there is a difference of 14.4 points on the visual analog scale (95% CI 8.5 to 20.4).

8.9 How to Describe the Test, the Statistical and Practical Significance of Your Findings in Your Report

8.9.1 Methods Section

In this section, you should set out the following:

- How your sample size was calculated. If it was not pre-calculated, say why not; maybe all available cases in a pre-existing database were used.
- The variable used to divide patients/institutions into two groups (e.g. laproscopic vs. abdominal surgical technique).
- The variable used to record the measured outcomes (e.g. the VAS pain score).
- The name of the statistical analysis employed (use the exact same wording as that in the menu structure of the package you used).
- Any options selected that differ from the program's default settings (e.g. the use of Welch's test in place of the classical t-test).
- The P-value that would be considered as statistically significant.
- The name of your statistical package along with its version number and supplier.

Suitable wording might be:

> A minimum sample size of 23 in each group was calculated using G*Power (v 3.1; Heinrich-Heine-Universität, Düsseldorf). The calculation was based on being able to detect a difference of 10 points between the mean pain scores for the two groups and a standard deviation of 10 points in both groups (*Give references or justification*). An a priori value of P <0.05 and a 90% power were used in the calculation. The main analysis was carried out using SPSS (Version 22; IBM Corporation), using the Independent-samples t-test.

8.9.2 Results Section

In this section, you should set out the following:

- The sample size, mean, and standard deviation for the outcome variable in each group, along with histograms or dot plots, dependent upon sample sizes.
- State if there was strong evidence of non-normality (giving the basis for the conclusion) and whether the standard deviations were approximately equal.

- If a switch was made to Welch's approximate t-test due to concerns about unequal standard deviations, this should be mentioned here.
- The P-value and a statement as to whether statistical significance was achieved.
- The difference between the group means, and its 95% confidence interval.

Suitable wording might be:

> A total of 30 participants were included in each group and their pain levels are summarized in Figure 8.2. The latter figure and normal probability plots showed no marked deviation from normal distributions. There was a statistically significant reduction (P-value <0.001) in pain scores experienced by those undergoing laparoscopic methods (40.8 ± 12.2) in comparison to those receiving the abdominal approach (55.2 ± 10.7). The difference between the mean pain levels was 14.4 points (95% confidence interval 8.5 to 20.37).

8.9.3 Discussion Section

It would be appropriate to explore the following points relating to your statistical analysis. Within this, you will need to provide and justify a value for the clinically/practically relevant difference.

- See Chapter 6 for guidance on interpreting statistically significant or non-significant results.
- Whether or not statistically significant – the implications for public policy or professional practice.

8.10 Relevant Videos etc.

The following are available at
www.wiley.com/go/Mackridge/APracticalApproachtoUsingStatisticsin HealthResearch

Videos

Video_1.1_SPSS_Basics: The absolute basics of using SPSS
Video_2.1_NormalityTesting: Using SPSS to determine whether measured data follows a normal distribution and log transformation to improve normality

Video_8.1_t-test_SampSize: Using G*Power to calculate necessary sample size for a t-test

Video_8.2_t-test: Using SPSS to perform the t-test and (if necessary) switch to Welch's test

SPSS data files

SPSS_8.1_Hysterectomies: The data for the example used to illustrate this chapter.

Spreadsheets

Spreadsheet_8.1_hysterectomies.xlsx: The data for the example used to illustrate this chapter.

9

Mann–Whitney Test

This test is also known as the "Wilcoxon rank sum test." However, that term is best avoided as it is so easily confused with the "Wilcoxon signed rank test."

9.1 When Is the Test Applied?

Figure 9.1 shows the circumstances where a Mann–Whitney test is used:

- The factor is categorical, with only **two** separate groups of individual patients or **two** sets of institutions etc.
- The outcome is an ordinal variable (or a continuously varying measured variable that is not normally distributed and cannot be transformed).
- Each participant provides just one outcome result – Participants A…E under condition 1 and F…J under condition 2.
- What is being tested is the appearance of generally higher values for the ordinal outcome under one condition than under the other.

Some examples are shown in Table 9.1. (For full details see Rowe Chapter 21, Section 2.)

9.2 An Example

In our example, we take the first case in Table 9.1. We have data on male and female clients' preferences for receiving stopping smoking

A Practical Approach to Using Statistics in Health Research: From Planning to Reporting, First Edition. Adam Mackridge and Philip Rowe.
© 2018 John Wiley & Sons, Inc. Published 2018 by John Wiley & Sons, Inc.
Companion website: www.wiley.com/go/Mackridge/
APracticalApproachtoUsingStatisticsinHealthResearch

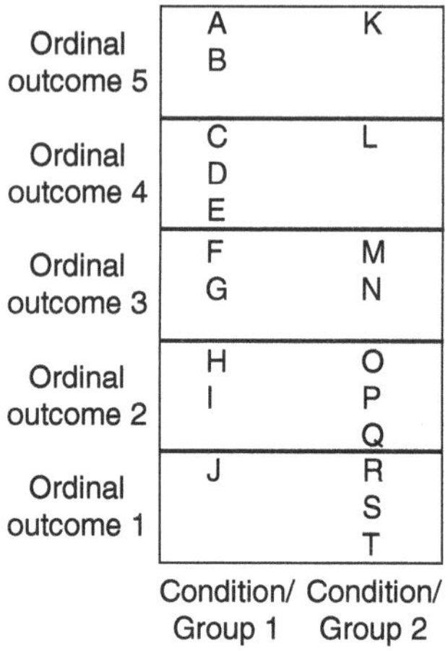

Figure 9.1 Circumstances when a Mann–Whitney test is used.

Table 9.1 Examples of studies that would be analyzed by a Mann–Whitney test.

Comparison made	Outcome	Question
Male versus female smokers	Agreement with the statement "I would prefer to get stopping smoking advice face-to-face rather than some other way." Five point scale: Strongly disagree (1); Disagree (2); Neutral (3); Agree (4); Strongly agree (5).	Is there a difference between the sexes in their preference for face-to-face stopping smoking advice over other forms of communication?
Patients randomized to receive or not receive acupuncture therapy prior to their dental treatment.	A ten-point dental anxiety score (high scores represent greatest anxiety).	Does acupuncture make any difference to patients' anxiety levels prior to dental treatment?
Children aged 11 to 16 living to the east versus those living west of a lead smelting plant. (Prevailing wind is west to east.)	Blood plasma concentration of lead. (Concentrations constitute continuous measured data, but the measurements are markedly non-normal and cannot be satisfactorily transformed to normality.)	Is there any difference between blood plasma concentrations of lead among children living downwind from the smelting plant compared to those living upwind?

advice in a face-to-face consultation, over other forms of advice. The dataset is available as either an MS Excel spreadsheet or an SPSS data file listed at the end of this chapter.

9.3 Presenting the Data

9.3.1 Numerically

You should report the numbers of individuals who select each of the five levels of outcome in both study groups. As explained in Chapter 3, there is no universally satisfactory way to summarize such data. A good starting point is the median and interquartile range, but the median may fail to demonstrate a contrast between your study groups even when a difference is quite clearly present. You may have to use the mean and SD in some cases, but this is best presented as an addition to the median rather than as a substitute.

For the current data set, the median scores are 2 for males (IQR = 2) and 3 for females (IQR = 1). Within our sample, males are less oriented toward personally provided advice.

9.3.2 Graphically

Bar charts such as Figure 9.2 are a good way to present this type of data. The tendency toward neutral or positive opinions among females compared to the preponderance of negative opinions among males is easily seen. A stacked bar chart could also be used.

9.3.3 Divide the Outcomes into Low and High Ranges

It may be appropriate to establish a cut-point to divide the data into low and high ranges. This is most defensible if this is already established practice with your particular scale or if there is a reasonable basis for choosing that cut-point. In the current case, we might want to focus on individuals who express some positive support for face-to-face delivery and so separate those expressing their agreement with the statement as levels 1, 2 or 3 (low values) from those at levels 4 or 5 (high). This would give 81 out of 171 (47%) high values among females and 45 out of 148 (30%) for the males.

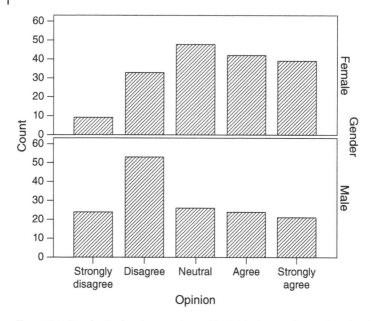

Figure 9.2 Bar charts showing numbers of individuals reporting various levels of agreement with the statement "I would prefer to get stopping smoking advice face-to-face rather than some other way" displayed by respondents' sex.

9.4 Data Requirements

9.4.1 Variables Required

With most statistics packages such as SPSS you will use two variables:

- A categorical variable (the factor) will be used to divide the participants into two groups: in our case, this describes participants' genders.
- An ordinal or continuous measured variable to record the outcome: in this case, their opinion scores. (In SPSS, you will have to declare the outcome as Scale even if it is actually ordinal. Otherwise the test will not be calculated.)

In some packages (such as Minitab) you will need to present the data in two variables, both containing values for the ordinal/measured endpoint (one for each gender).

9.4.2   Normal Distributions and Equality of Standard Deviations

This is a nonparametric test, so there are no requirements for normal distributions or equal standard deviations.

9.4.3   Equal Sample Sizes

Equality of sample sizes is not a condition for this test; they are unequal in the current example. However, for any given total number of observations, statistical power is greatest with the data divided as equally as possible between the two samples.

9.5   An Outline of the Test

Three aspects of the data will determine whether your results are statistically significant:

- The extent of the contrast between the outcomes. If one group produces markedly higher values than the other, significance is likely. Marginal differences are less likely to achieve significance.
- Widely varying scores within each study group are less likely to result in significance than consistent values.
- The size of your samples: It is very difficult for small samples to provide adequate evidence of a real difference, whereas large samples are more likely to achieve statistical significance.

9.6   Statistical Significance

For the current example, the data is statistically significant ($P<0.001$).

9.7   Planning Sample Sizes

An exact calculation of necessary sample sizes for a study to be analyzed by the Mann–Whitney test is not straightforward; it would include specification of the data distribution anticipated within both study groups. As you have selected a nonparametric test, you are probably not anticipating that your samples will follow simple normal distributions.

A pragmatic approach can be based upon the fact that even with the most unfavorable possible data distribution, the power of a Mann–Whitney test can only fall to 86% of the power you would achieve by applying a t-test to the same data. Taking this approach, you can calculate sample sizes that would be required for a t-test and then add 15%. This will give adequate sample sizes (probably generous) when you apply a Mann–Whitney test to the results.

See a video listed at the end of this chapter for instructions on using G*Power to calculate sample sizes for a t-test.

9.8 Carrying Out the Test

See a video listed at the end of this chapter for instructions on using SPSS to carry out the Mann–Whitney test.

9.9 Describing the Effect Size

There are several possible approaches to describing the extent of the difference between the two groups. No single one is applicable in all cases. You need to consider what is appropriate for your particular study.

- Report the difference between the median values for the two groups. Where the range of possible rankings is small, this may be a very crude indicator of difference and can sometimes be zero, i.e. equal medians for the two groups despite a histogram and the Mann–Whitney test indicating a clear and statistically significant difference.
- If the difference between medians is too insensitive to illustrate your findings, additionally report the difference between the mean values for the two groups. Quote the insensitivity of the median as justification for the additional use of the mean.
- Contrast the proportion of individuals in the two study groups who report values above/below a critical level. In the current case, 47% versus 30% respectively of females and males expressing Agreement or Strong agreement with the statement.

9.10 How to Report the Test

9.10.1 Methods Section

In this section, you should set out the following:

- How your sample size was calculated. (If it was not pre-calculated, say why not; maybe all available cases in a pre-existing database were used.)
- The variable used to divide patients/institutions into two groups.
- The variable used to record the ordinal or continuous measured outcome.
- The name of the statistical analysis employed (use the exact same wording as that in the menu structure of the package you used).
- Any options selected if these differ from the program's defaults.
- The P-value that would be considered as statistically significant.
- The name of your statistical package along with its version number and supplier.

Suitable wording might be:

> The minimum sample size was calculated as 125 in each group, using the approach described by Mackridge & Rowe (2018). In this, a difference of 0.5 (or more) between the two mean scores was to be detectable (*give references or justification*), and it was assumed that the standard deviation among the scores would be 1.30 points in both study groups. The a priori P-value was set as <0.05, and 80% power was used in the calculation. The calculation was carried out using G*Power (Heinrich-Heine-Universität, Düsseldorf).
>
> The scores for the two genders were compared via the Mann–Whitney test using SPSS (Version 23; IBM Corporation).

9.10.2 Results Section

In this section, you should set out the following:

- The number of participants in each study group.
- A table or bar charts presenting the numbers selecting each level of agreement for each group separately.
- A measure of effect size – one of the following:
  - the median and interquartile range for both genders; or
  - (possibly) the mean and SD for both genders; or

- the proportions of males and females who agreed or strongly agreed.
- If the original data was continuous measured, describe its distribution and state why a nonparametric test was used.
- The P-value for the test and a statement as to whether the result was statistically significant.

Suitable wording might be

> A total of 148 males and 171 females responded to the question about preference for face-to-face stopping-smoking advice, and Figure 9.2 shows the numbers in each group expressing various levels of agreement with the statement. Levels of agreement with the statement were statistically significantly (P<0.001) higher among females than males. The proportions expressing agreement or strong agreement were 47% for females and 30% for males.

9.10.3   Discussion Section

A key part of your discussion will be to compare the effect size seen in your work against the minimum clinically/practically relevant difference. You will need to provide and justify a value for the latter.

Nonparametric methods do not generate any easily used confidence interval for the effect size, so you will not be able to follow fully the recommendations in Chapter 6. Some suggestions follow.

- For a non-significant result: If sample sizes are small, be wary of saying there is no effect; one may be present but you have failed to detect it. With large samples, you can more safely say that there is either no effect or, at the very least, any effect is very small and therefore probably not of any practical relevance.
- For a significant result: Discuss whether the effect size is great enough to be of practical consequence, and its implications for public policy or professional practice.

Rowe (2015, Section 21.2.5)[1] discusses in detail the interpretation of a statistically significant finding with a nonparametric test. It is always safe to use wording such as "Values for the endpoint are higher in

---

[1] Rowe P. Essential statistics for the pharmaceutical sciences, 2nd edn. Chichester: Wiley, 2015.

group A than in group B." Any claim that the median or mean is higher in one group than in the other would only be reliable if the distributions of the two sets of data were appropriate.

9.11 Relevant Videos etc.

The following are available at
www.wiley.com/go/Mackridge/APracticalApproachtoUsingStatistics inHealthResearch

Videos

Video_1.1_SPSS_Basics: The absolute basics of using SPSS
Video_8.1_G*Power_t-test: Using G*Power for t-test sample size calculation
Video_9.1_MannWhitneyTest: Using SPSS for the Mann–Whitney test

SPSS data files

SPSS_9.1_SmokingAdvice: The data for the example used to illustrate this chapter.

Spreadsheets

Spreadsheet_9.1_SmokingAdvice: The data for the example used to illustrate this chapter.

10

One-Way Analysis of Variance (ANOVA) – Including Dunnett's and Tukey's Follow Up Tests

10.1   When Is the Test Applied?

Figure 10.1 shows the circumstances where a one-way analysis of variance (ANOVA) is used:

- The factor is categorical with **three or more** different conditions or categories.
- The outcome is a continuous measured variable.
- Each subject provides just one outcome result – in Figure 10.1, Subjects A...E under condition 1, F...J under condition 2 and so on.
- The question is whether there are differences among the mean values of the measured outcome under the various conditions.

Some examples of studies where ANOVA would be appropriate are shown in Table 10.1. (For full details, see Rowe (2015) chapter 14, sections 1 and 2.)

10.2   An Example

In our example, we take the last case in Table 10.1. Do either of the two dietary modifications change the mean blood cholesterol levels compared to the control condition – Group (a)? The dataset is available as an SPSS data file or MS Excel spreadsheet as listed at the end of this chapter.

A Practical Approach to Using Statistics in Health Research: From Planning to Reporting, First Edition. Adam Mackridge and Philip Rowe.
Companion website: www.wiley.com/go/Mackridge/
APracticalApproachtoUsingStatisticsinHealthResearch

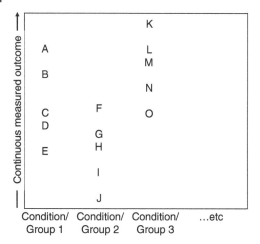

Figure 10.1 Structure of an experiment or survey where a one-way analysis of variance would be appropriate.

10.3 Presenting the Data

10.3.1 Numerically

You should report the sample size, mean, and standard deviation for the measured outcome in each of the study groups.

10.3.2 Graphically

With large amounts of data, histograms work well, but for smaller datasets you may have to use some form of dot plot. In the current case, there is enough data for histograms to work satisfactorily, and Figure 10.2 shows trends toward reduced circulating cholesterol levels with both the margarine and nut supplementation, whereas the controls have changes centered close to zero.

10.4 Data Requirements

10.4.1 Variables Required

You will use two variables (columns in SPSS):

- A categorical variable will divide the subjects into groups: in our case, this describes the type of dietary change.

- A continuous measured variable will contain the outcome: the individual changes in cholesterol levels during the three month study period.

10.4.2 Normality of Distribution for the Outcome Variable Within the Three Samples

It is a requirement for ANOVA that the data within each study group should form an approximate normal distribution. See Sections 2.2.1

Table 10.1 Examples of studies that would be analyzed by a one-way analysis of variance.

Comparison made	Outcome	Question
Four groups of women using different birth control methods - Combined oral contraceptive - Progestogen only oral contraceptive - Intramuscular injectable progestogen - Intrauterine device	Change in body weight (kg) during first three months of use	Are there any differences in mean weight change with different methods of contraception?
Subjects separated according to blood group (O, A, B, or AB)	Blood concentration of thrombomodulin (a circulating anticoagulant protein)	Do mean levels of this anticoagulant differ according to blood group?
Patients with chronic back pain a) Trained in progressive muscle relaxation b) Undergoing cognitive behavioral therapy c) Control group receiving "treatment as usual"	Change in visual analog scale (VAS) for pain (100 point scale)	Are there any differences in changes in perceived pain levels among the three treatment groups?
Three groups of subjects who for a three month period: a) Make no dietary change b) Use a cholesterol lowering spread (margarine) in place of their normal spread c) Supplement their diets with 35 g of nuts per day	Change in serum cholesterol between beginning and end of study period	Do the experimental spread or additional nuts change mean serum cholesterol levels?

Figure 10.2 Histograms of changes in blood cholesterol levels (mmol/l) over the three month study period for participants (a) making no dietary change, (b) using a cholesterol lowering spread in place of their normal spread, and (c) adding 35 g of nuts per day to their diet.

and 2.2.2 for details of how to check for non-normal distribution and possible transformations to normality. In our case, Figure 10.2 showed no evidence of non-normal distribution in any of the three datasets[1]:

- The data are unimodal.
- The highest frequencies are near the middle of the range of values (no evidence of skewness).
- Normal probability plots of this data show no signs of long-tailed distributions.

Notice that you must check for normality in each dataset separately. If the various study groups are all normally distributed but have different means, then a combination of all the datasets will not be normally distributed.

In the absence of any of the problems mentioned in Section 2.2.1, you can probably treat the data as adequately approximating normal distributions. If the data cannot be transformed to normality, you can instead use the Kruskal–Wallis test (Chapter 11). See a video listed at the end of this chapter for details of using computer packages to check for normality and methods for transforming non-normal data to normality.

10.4.3 Standard Deviations

It is also a requirement for ANOVA that all your samples should have similar standard deviations (SDs) (See Section 6.1). If your SDs look markedly different (e.g. one SD twice as great as another), there is a variant form of ANOVA (Welch's) that will tolerate such differences. However, with approximately similar SDs, it is best to use the classical ANOVA as it is a little more powerful. A video listed at the end of this chapter shows how to switch to Welch's test.

---

[1] Note that in our example, we have recorded cholesterol measurements at the start and end of the study period and used these to calculate each individual participant's cholesterol change. Since it is the *changes* that form the study outcome, these values are what need to be normally distributed – there is no need for the initial and final cholesterol values to form normal distributions.

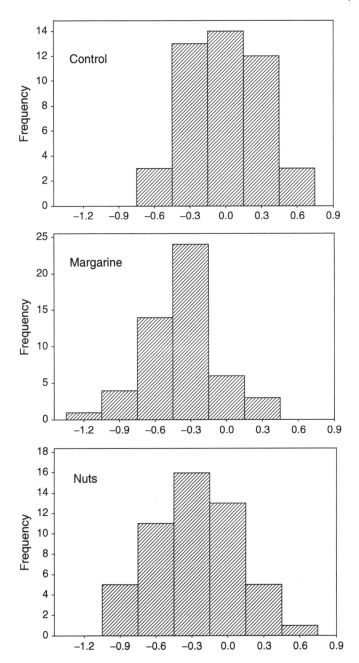

10.4.4 Sample Sizes

Equality of sample sizes is **not** a condition for this test. However, for any given total number of observations, statistical power is greatest with the data divided equally among the groups. The only exception to this rule arises if you intend to use a Dunnett's follow up test (See Section 10.6). This test makes increased use of the data from the reference group, and it is useful to have a larger sample size for this group when using Dunnett's follow up test.

10.5 An Outline of the Test

Three aspects of the data will determine whether your results are statistically significant:

- The differences **between** the means for the various groups/conditions: Large differences are more likely to be judged statistically significant than small ones.
- The standard deviation **within** each sample: Highly varying data reduces the chances of significance.
- The size of your samples: Large samples are more likely to achieve significance than small ones.

10.6 Follow Up Tests

A significant result from the ANOVA tells you that at least one of the group means differs from one of the others to a statistically significant degree. Very frequently, this is not particularly useful in itself: you want to know exactly which condition/group differs from which other. So-called "Follow up" tests are used to answer this question. There are huge numbers of these "Follow up" tests available, but the following two will cover most situations:

- Dunnett's test: This takes one group as a base-line reference; this would typically be your control group (treatment as usual or placebo intervention). It then tests for differences between the reference group and all other groups in turn. If there are groups A, B, and C and A is treated as the reference, then tests will be made of

A versus B and of A versus C. No test will be made for any difference between B and C.

- Tukey's test: This tests for differences between all possible pairs of groups and does not require a reference group, so is likely to be more appropriate when you do not have a control group within your study design. If there are groups A, B, and C, it will test for differences between A and B, between A and C, and between B and C.

The output from these tests will include confidence intervals for the size of the differences between the means for all pairs of groups considered.

It is important to note that follow up tests typically require increased sample sizes where there are larger numbers of groups to compare. It is therefore important not to introduce additional study groups beyond those necessitated by the research question. A fuller account of the theory of these tests is presented in Rowe (2015) section 14.2.6.[1]

Details of how to perform ANOVA and how to add follow up tests are covered in a video listed at the end of this chapter.

10.7 Planning Sample Sizes

As calculating the sample size for ANOVA in G*Power is complex and burdensome, we do not recommend using it. Below is a simpler approach that will provide you with the bare minimum requirement for your sample size, based on some key details of your study design:

1) How many different study groups will be considered?
2) The anticipated difference between the mean values for the two study groups that will show the greatest difference.
3) The anticipated standard deviation within the various groups. (See Section 6.2).
4) The power you wish to achieve – see glossary – we have assumed the commonly used figure of 90%.

---

[1] Rowe P. Essential statistics for the pharmaceutical sciences, 2nd edn. Chichester: Wiley, 2015.

Table 10.2 Necessary sample sizes per group for a one-way analysis of variance requiring 90% power.

Ratio of greatest difference to SD	Three groups	Four groups	Five groups	Six groups
0.1	2532	2836	3082	3295
0.2	634	710	772	825
0.3	283	316	344	367
0.4	160	179	194	207
0.5	103	115	125	133
0.6	72	80	87	93
0.7	53	59	64	69
0.8	41	46	50	53
0.9	33	36	39	42
1.0	27	30	32	34
1.25	18	20	21	23
1.5	13	14	15	16
2	8	9	9	10

You then calculate the ratio of (2) to (3) from the list (Difference in means/Standard deviation) and use this, along with your answer to (1) to select the relevant figure from Table 10.2.

For the current example, we have anticipated that the cholesterol reducing spread and control groups will provide the greatest contrast, with the spread causing a mean reduction of 0.25 mmol/l compared to no change in the mean for the control group. This gives a between-group contrast of 0.25 mmol/l. We have determined from previous studies that the SD for all groups is likely be 0.30 mmol/l. The ratio is then 0.25/0.30 = 0.83. From Table 10.2, three study groups and a ratio of 0.80 would require a sample size of 41. As our ratio falls between 0.8 and 0.9, we can reasonably round this down to 40 in each study group.

10.8   Carrying Out the Test

See a video listed at the end of this chapter for detailed instructions on using SPSS to carry out an ANOVA and follow up tests.

10.9   Describing the Effect Size

Effect sizes are best described as the differences between means (plus 95% confidence intervals) for whatever pairs of groups are considered in the follow up test.

10.10   How to Report the Test

10.10.1   Methods

Within your report you should specify:

- How your sample size was calculated. (If it was not pre-calculated, say why not; maybe all available cases in a pre-existing database were used.)
- Which groups were compared and the particular characteristic that defines the groups.
- The continuously varying end-point.
- The name of the statistical test employed and that of any follow up test used (use the exact same wording as that in the menu structure of the software package you used).
- Any options selected other than the defaults within the package used and the reasons for this (e.g. Using Welch's version of the test if SDs are severely unequal).
- The P-value that would be considered as statistically significant.
- The name of your statistical package along with its version number and supplier.

Suitable wording could be:

> Minimum sample sizes were calculated as 40 per group, using the approach described in Mackridge & Rowe (2018), based on a predicted intergroup difference of 0.25 mmol/L (*give references or justification*), a standard deviation of 0.3 mmol/L (*references or justification*), and a power of 90%. An a priori P value of <0.05 was set.
>
> A One-Way ANOVA was performed using SPSS (Version 23; IBM Corporation) comparing cholesterol changes in the three dietary groups. A Dunnett's test treating the control as the reference group was also undertaken to further explore intergroup differences.

10.10.2   Results Section

In this section, you should set out the following:

- The number of participants/cases in each study group.
- The mean and standard deviation for the end-point in each group along with histograms or dot plots, dependent upon sample sizes.
- State whether there was strong evidence of non-normality.
- If a switch was made to Welch's alternative form of the test due to concerns about unequal standard deviations, this should be described.
- The value of the test-statistic (F) for ANOVA is frequently reported, but its usefulness is questionable and it is better omitted. However, the P-value would certainly be reported.
- Whether statistical significance was achieved for the overall ANOVA.
- Whether the comparisons within any follow up test were statistically significant.
- The differences (plus confidence intervals) between the means for each pair of groups compared in any follow up test.

Suitable wording might be:

> There were a total of 148 participants in the study, with 45 in the control group, 52 using margarine, and 51 using nuts. Histograms of the results showed no evidence of non-normal data distributions. The mean ±SD for the change in cholesterol levels between the baseline and 3 months were Control −0.011±0.333; Margarine −0.365±0.306; and Nuts −0.282±0.347. An ANOVA demonstrated statistically significant differences between the study groups (P<0.001) and a Dunnett's test confirmed that both intervention groups had statistically significant reduced cholesterol levels compared to the controls. Differences between the mean responses for the control and margarine groups were −0.354 mmol/l (CI −0.205 to −0.503; P<0.001) and between the control and nuts groups were -0.271 mmol/l (CI −0.121 to −0.421; P<0.001).

10.10.3   Discussion Section

It would be appropriate to explore the following points relating to your statistical analysis. Within this, you will need to provide and justify a value for the clinically/practically relevant difference between any two groups.

- See Sections 6.5 and 6.6 for guidance on interpreting statistically significant or non-significant results.
- Whether or not statistically significant – the implications for public policy or professional practice.

10.11   Relevant Videos etc.

The following are available at
www.wiley.com/go/Mackridge/APracticalApproachtoUsingStatisticsin
HealthResearch

Videos

Video_1.1_SPSS_Basics: The absolute basics of using SPSS
Video_2.1_Normality testing: Using SPSS to determine whether measured data follows a normal distribution and log transformation to improve normality
Video_10_1_ANOVA: Using SPSS to perform a one-way analysis of variance and follow up tests and switching to the Welch test where necessary.

SPSS data files

SPSS_10.1_Cholesterol: The data for the example used to illustrate this chapter.

Spreadsheets

Spreadsheet_10.1_Cholesterol: The data for the example used to illustrate this chapter.

11

Kruskal–Wallis

11.1   When Is the Test Applied?

Figure 11.1 shows the circumstances where a Kruskal–Wallis test is used:

- There are a number of categorically different conditions or groups. Three are indicated in the figure, but there could be more than this.
- The outcome is an ordinal variable (or a continuously varying measured variable that is not normally distributed). Five levels of the ordinal measure are shown in the figure, but it could be more (or less) than this.
- Each participant provides just one outcome result – Participants A-H under condition 1, I-P under condition 2, and so on.
- What are being tested are the apparently greater or lower values of the ordinal outcome under the various conditions.

Some examples of studies where the Kruskal–Wallis test is applicable are shown in Table 11.1. (For a more detailed description of this test, see Rowe (2015) section 21.4.2.)

11.2   An Example

In our example, we take the last case in Table 11.1: Experience of menstrual problems with various forms of contraception. The extent of any problems was expressed on a five-point ordinal scale of 1 = Nothing of concern; 2 = Slight; 3 = Moderate; 4 = Problematic; 5 = Severe.

A Practical Approach to Using Statistics in Health Research: From Planning to Reporting, First Edition. Adam Mackridge and Philip Rowe.
© 2018 John Wiley & Sons, Inc. Published 2018 by John Wiley & Sons, Inc.
Companion website: www.wiley.com/go/Mackridge/
APracticalApproachtoUsingStatisticsinHealthResearch

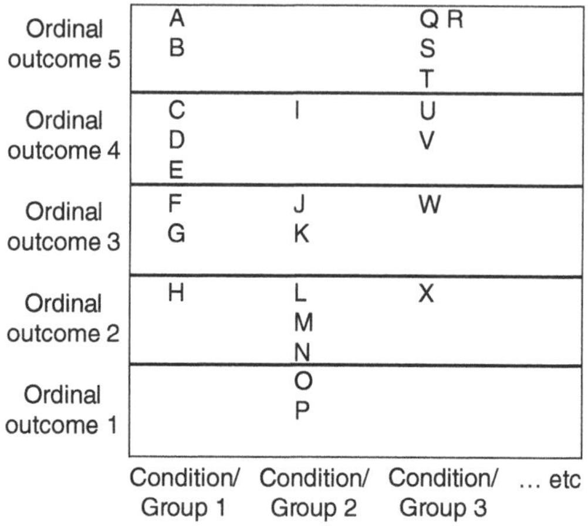

Figure 11.1 The structure of a study suitable for analysis by a Kruskal–Wallis test.

The dataset is available in SPSS and MS Excel formats as listed at the end of this chapter.

11.3 Presenting the Data

11.3.1 Numerically

You could tabulate the numbers of individuals who report each of the five levels of menstrual problems in each study group as in Table 11.2.

As explained in Chapter 3, the median for five-point scales is notoriously insensitive. Despite the marked difference between progestogen only OCs and IUDs shown in Figure 11.2, their medians are identical. Consequently, it would be appropriate in this case to follow the advice in Section 3.2.1 and make additional use of the mean and SD (See Table 11.3) as this better illustrates the contrast between the progestogen only OC and IUDs, and is useful in describing this data clearly.

Another way to summarize the data is to present the proportions in each group with values above/below some sensible cut-off value. If we consider that experiencing a moderate problem (or worse) brings a significant risk that the woman might want to discontinue use of the method, then we could use this as a cut point (see Table 11.4).

Table 11.1 Examples of studies that would be analyzed by a Kruskal–Wallis test.

Comparison made	Outcome	Question
Three groups: Senior and junior nurses and final year nursing students.	Score on a knowledge test containing eight questions concerning analgesics.	Are there different levels of knowledge among the three groups?
Families classified into three groups based on parental education level: Low, medium, and high.	Number of decayed, missing, or filled teeth in children aged thirteen. (Data very non-normal)	Does children's dental health vary according to parental education levels?
Three groups of residents: Inner city, suburban, and rural.	Daily sugar consumption. (Data is continuous measured, but results show varying degrees of positive skew – i.e. non-normal distribution)	Does sugar consumption vary according to type of residential area?
Four groups of women (aged 30-35) using different birth control methods • Combined oral contraceptive • Progestogen only oral contraceptive • Intramuscular injectable progestogen • Copper containing intrauterine device (IUD).	Response to the question "To what extent do you suffer from irregular, painful, or heavy menstrual periods or intermenstrual bleeding?" Responses on a five-point scale.	Does experience of irregular, painful, or heavy menstrual periods or intermenstrual bleeding vary with different methods of contraception?

11.3.2 Graphically

Stacked bar charts such as Figure 11.2 are often a good way to present this type of data. They show the greater proportions of the higher levels of problems (moderate, problematic, or severe) with the progestogen only OC and injectables, and the generally low levels of problems for the combined OC group. This graph only presents proportions, not absolute numbers, so you would also need to include the numbers in each study group for clarity of reporting.

Table 11.2 Number of women reporting various levels of menstrual problems with different forms of contraception.

	Experience of menstrual problems				
	(1) Nothing of concern	(2) Slight	(3) Moderate	(4) Problematic	(5) Severe
Combined OC	95	24	11	5	0
Progestogen only OC	30	39	40	8	4
Injectable	29	43	24	6	1
IUD	49	40	19	3	0

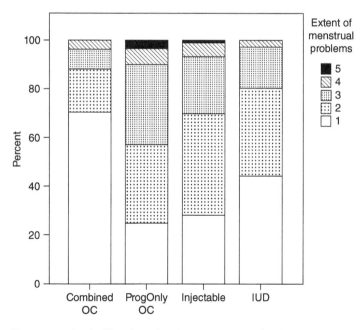

Figure 11.2 Stacked bar chart showing percentages of individuals reporting various levels of menstrual problems displayed by contraceptive type. Higher grades indicate greater problems.

Table 11.3 Descriptive statistics for levels of menstrual problems in women using different methods of contraception.

	Sample size	Median	Interquartile range	Mean	SD
Combined OC	135	1	1	1.45	0.80
Progestogen only OC	121	2	1.5	2.31	1.03
Injectable	103	2	2	2.10	0.91
IUD	111	2	1	1.78	0.82

Table 11.4 Numbers (and percentages) of women reporting lower or higher levels of menstrual problems with different forms of contraception.

	Nothing of concern or slight issues	Moderate to severe problems
Combined OC	119 (88%)	16 (12%)
Progestogen only OC	69 (57%)	52 (43%)
Injectable	72 (70%)	31 (30%)
IUD	89 (80%)	22 (20%)

11.4 Data Requirements

11.4.1 Variables Required

With almost all statistics packages, you will use two variables (columns in SPSS):

- A categorical variable will be used to divide the participants into groups: in our case, this describes the four contraception types.
- An ordinal or continuous measured variable to record the outcome: in this case, the five menstrual problem values. (In SPSS, you will have to declare the outcome as Scale even if it is actually ordinal. Otherwise the test will not be calculated.)

11.4.2 Normal Distributions and Standard Deviations

This is a nonparametric test and so there is no requirement for normal distributions or equal standard deviations in the data sets.

11.4.3 Equal Sample Sizes

Equal sample sizes are not needed for this test (they are unequal in the current example). However, for any given total number of observations, statistical power is greatest with the data is divided equally between the various groups.

11.5 An Outline of the Test

Three aspects of the data will determine whether your results are statistically significant:

- The extent of the differences **between** the groups. If one group produces markedly higher values than one of the others, significance is likely. Marginal differences are less likely to achieve significance.
- Widely varying values **within** each study group are less likely to result in significance than cases with consistent values within each group.
- The size of your samples: It is very difficult for small samples to provide enough evidence of a real difference, whereas large samples are more likely to achieve statistical significance.

11.6 Planning Sample Sizes

An exact calculation of necessary sample sizes for a study to be analyzed by a Kruskal–Wallis test is not straightforward. However, a pragmatic approach can be based upon the fact that even with the most unfavorable circumstances, the power of a Kruskal–Wallis test is 86% of that achieved by applying a one-way analysis of variance (ANOVA) to the same data. Taking this approach, you can follow the procedure set out in Section 10.7 and then add 15% to the number. This will give adequate sample sizes when you apply a Kruskal–Wallis test to the results.

11.7 Carrying Out the Test

See a video listed at the end of the chapter for detailed instructions on using SPSS to carry out the Kruskal–Wallis test.

11.8   Describing the Effect Size

There are several possible approaches to describing the extent of the difference between the groups, and no single one is applicable in all cases. You should review the discussion in Section 11.3 and consider what is appropriate for your particular study. The main options are:

- Report the difference between the median values for any pair of groups that is of interest; however this can be very insensitive.
- Additionally, report the difference between the mean values for two groups. Use the inadequate sensitivity of the medians to justify the inclusion of the means.
- Contrast the proportion of individuals in the study groups who report values above/below a critical level (See Table 11.4).

11.9   Determining Which Group Differs from Which Other

As with ANOVA, just knowing that there are some differences between the groups may well not be adequate; you may want to know which pairs of groups differ. The Kruskal–Wallis test does not have any simple equivalents of the Tukey or Dunnett's tests (See Chapter 10). The best (albeit imperfect) solution is to carry out repeated Mann–Whitney tests between whichever pairs of groups you consider to be of interest, but apply the Bonferroni correction (Section 5.2.3) in order to avoid inflating the risk of false positives. If you wished to test every possible pair of groups in this study, that would entail a total of six tests, and the Bonferroni correction would require $P < 0.0083$ for any claim of statistical significance. In the current case, five of the six possible comparisons are statistically significant ($P < 0.001$) with just the progestogen only OCs vs injectables ($P = 0.111$) and injectables vs IUDs ($P = 0.010$) not reaching significance.

11.10   How to Report the Test

11.10.1   Methods Section

- How your sample size was calculated. (If it was not pre-calculated, say why not.)

- The variable used to divide patients/organizations into groups (the factor).
- The variable used to record the ordinal or continuous measured outcome.
- The name of the statistical analysis employed (use the exact same wording as that in the package you used).
- Any options selected that differ from the program's defaults.
- The P-value that would be considered as statistically significant.
- The name of your statistical package along with its version number and supplier.

Suitable wording might be:

> Minimum sample sizes of 100 per group were calculated using the method described by Mackridge and Rowe (2018). This was based on assumptions that a difference of 0.5 between the mean values for two of the groups should be detectable (*give references or justification*), that the standard deviation among the values would be 0.8 in all study groups (*references or justification*), and that statistical significance would require a P value of <0.05 and the target power would be 90%.
>
> Overall statistical significance was assessed using the Kruskal–Wallis test and then, as follow up tests, all possible pairs of groups were compared using Mann–Whitney tests, applying a Bonferroni corrected requirement for $P < 0.0083$ for a claim of statistical significance. Both these tests were implemented using SPSS (Version 23; IBM Corporation).

11.10.2 Results Section

In this section, you should set out the following:

- The number of participants in each study group.
- With ordinal outcome data, a table or bar chart presenting the numbers reporting each level of the ordinal scale, for each group separately.
- A summary measure that can be used to assess the effect size (see Section 11.8).
- If the original data was continuous measured, describe its distribution and state why a nonparametric test was used.
- The P-value for the test and a statement as to whether the result was statistically significant.
- If follow up tests were performed, describe these.

Suitable wording might be:

> A total of 470 women participated in the study, with 135 receiving combined OC, 121 Progestogen only OC, 103 injectable contraception and 111 having an IUD fitted. A Kruskal–Wallis test showed statistically significant differences (P < 0.001) among the levels of menstrual problems in the various groups (See Figure 11.2). Bonferroni corrected Mann–Whitney tests showed statistically significant contrasts between all possible pairs of groups (P < 0.001) except the pairing of progestogen only OCs and injectables (P = 0.111) and injectables and IUDs (P = 0.010). The proportions of women describing problems as Moderate (or worse) in each group were: Combined OC 12%; Progestogen only OC 43%; Injectables 30%; IUD 20%.

11.10.3 Discussion Section

A key part of your discussion will be to compare any effect sizes seen in your work against the minimum clinically/practically relevant difference. You will need to provide and justify a value for the latter.

Nonparametric methods do not generate any easily used confidence interval for the effect size, so you will not be able to follow fully the recommendations in Chapter 6. Some suggestions follow.

- For a non-significant result: If sample sizes are small, be wary of saying there is no effect; one may be present, but you have failed to detect it. Where your sample has exceeded your calculated required sample size and the variance (SD) is no larger than that used in your calculation, you can more safely say that there is either no effect or, at the very least, any effect is very small (less than the minimum your set out in your sample size calculation) and therefore unlikely to be of any practical relevance.
- For a significant result: Discuss whether the effect size is great enough to be of practical consequence and its implications for public policy or professional practice.

Rowe (2015, section 21.2.5)[1] discusses in detail the interpretation of a statistically significant finding with a nonparametric test. It is always safe to use wording such as "Values for the endpoint are higher in group

---

[1] Rowe P. Essential statistics for the pharmaceutical sciences, 2nd edn. Chichester: Wiley, 2015.

A than in group B." Any claim that the median or mean is higher in one group than in the other would only be reliable if the distributions of the two sets of data conformed to the appropriate requirements.

11.11   Relevant Videos etc.

The following are available at www.wiley.com/go/Mackridge/APracticalApproachtoUsingStatisticsin HealthResearch

Videos

Video_1.1_SPSS_Basics: The absolute basics of using SPSS
Video _11.1_Kruskal–Wallis: Using SPSS to perform a Kruskal–Wallis analysis

SPSS data files

SPSS_11.1_Contraception: The data for the example used to illustrate this chapter.

Spreadsheets

Spreadsheet_11.1_Contraception.xlsx: The data for the example used to illustrate this chapter.

12

McNemar's Test

12.1 When Is the Test Applied?

Figure 12.1 shows the circumstances where McNemar's test is used:

- The factor is categorical with **two** different study conditions.
- The outcome is categorical with **two** possible options.
- All participants provide outcome results under **both** study conditions.
- Subjects A, B, G, and H show no change in outcome as they move from condition 1 to 2, but for subjects C…F, the change in conditions does produce a change in outcome. What is being tested is the apparently greater tendency to change from outcome A to B than from B to A.

(For full details, see Rowe (2015), section 18.6)

Note that this test can also be used with matched pairs. In Figure 12.1, "A" might refer to two matched individuals with one individual studied under one set of circumstances and the other under the alternative conditions. See the final two examples in Table 12.1.

Some examples where McNemar's test would be appropriate are shown in Table 12.1.

12.2 An Example

In the first example (Table 12.1), each respondent fills in a questionnaire that ostensibly concerns participation in sporting activity, but includes a question as to whether they have ever smoked cannabis. They also take part in a face-to-face interview on sport that includes

A Practical Approach to Using Statistics in Health Research: From Planning to Reporting,
First Edition. Adam Mackridge and Philip Rowe.
© 2018 John Wiley & Sons, Inc. Published 2018 by John Wiley & Sons, Inc.
Companion website: www.wiley.com/go/Mackridge/
APracticalApproachtoUsingStatisticsinHealthResearch

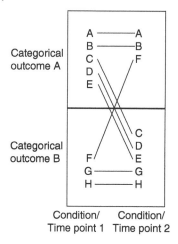

Figure 12.1 Structure of a study where a McNemar's test would be used.

this question. The point of interest is whether people are more likely to acknowledge drug use in one context relative to the other. Note that the data is "related" or "paired" as we have two responses from each participant. The dataset is available as an MS Excel spreadsheet or an SPSS data file listed at the end of this chapter.

12.3 Presenting the Data

The most effective way to present the data is as in Table 12.2. This preserves the paired nature of the data and, in particular, the reader can identify the key individuals whose responses were different according to the means of questioning.

12.4 Data Requirements

You will need two categorical variables (columns in SPSS).

- One will record each participant's response within the questionnaire.
- The other will record each participant's responses during the interview.
- Each row represents one participant's responses (with matched pairs, you would record the outcomes for each participant in a pair within the same row).

Table 12.1 Examples of studies that would be analyzed by McNemar's test.

Comparison made	Outcome	Question
Participants asked in a questionnaire if they have ever used cannabis and asked again in a face-to-face interview.	Do/Do not admit to use	Does the context influence the likelihood of admitting to cannabis use?
Patients with Type II diabetes carry out self-monitoring of blood glucose before and again after receiving written instructions on correct procedure.	Do/Do not make at least one mistake during the procedure	Does receipt of the written instructions change the risk of making an error?
Pairs of matched individuals in addiction treatment program maintained over six months, with one of each pair being provided with methadone and the other being supplied with diamorphine.	Do/Do not achieve an acceptable level of attendance during that period of treatment	Does supplying diamorphine alter the likelihood of adequate attendance?
Pairs of patients matched according to sex, age, and level of educational achievement. One patient from each pair trained to use an inhaler by a nurse and the other trained by a doctor.	Satisfactory or unsatisfactory technique for inhaler use	Are those trained by one professional group more successful than those trained by the other?

Table 12.2 Responses to the question "Have you ever smoked cannabis?" when posed as part of a questionnaire or in a face-to-face interview.

	Answered "No" in questionnaire	Answered "Yes" in questionnaire
Answered "No" in face-to-face interview	313	43
Answered "Yes" in face-to-face interview	6	112

12.5 An Outline of the Test

This test distinguishes between responses that are "Concordant" (where the outcome is the same in both conditions) and "Discordant" (where the outcome changes in different settings). In Table 12.2 there are 313 concordant No responses and 112 concordant Yes responses, respectively. Meanwhile, there are 43 discordant responses with an answer of Yes only in the questionnaire and 6 discordant cases with an answer of Yes only in the interview. The outcome of the test depends only on whether the two discordant figures are convincingly different; the size of the concordant sets is irrelevant.

12.6 Planning Sample Sizes

You will need the following values:

1) An estimate of the proportion of individuals who will give discordant responses in one of the possible directions. For our example, we have predicted that 2% will answer yes in the interview and no in the questionnaire.
2) An estimate of the proportion of individuals who will give discordant responses in the other possible direction. For our example, we have predicted that 10% will answer yes in the questionnaire and no in the interview.
3) You can then calculate the ratio of (1) to (2) as a measure of the sensitivity you require. Based on our predictions, of 10% and 2%, we wish to be able to detect a ratio between the two patterns of discordant response of 5.0. Note that smaller ratios will require much larger sample sizes, and restricting yourself to detecting ratios well above or below 1 will allow smaller sample sizes.
4) The power you require (see glossary) – we have used 90% in our example as this is suitable for most purposes.
5) What P-value[1] you will consider as statistically significant. Typically, P-values of less than 0.05 are used.

Ideally, the figures for (1) and (2) would come from published work or a pilot study. If this is not possible, you would need to provide a justification in your write-up as to how you estimated these figures.

---

[1] The p-value may be referred to in software packages as "Alpha" – see glossary.

A spreadsheet for calculation of necessary sample size and a video demonstrating its use are listed at the end of this chapter.

12.7 Carrying Out the Test

The data will probably be presented in two variables (columns in SPSS):

- One recording the first result for each participant.
- One for the participants' second results.

Each participant (or pair of participants) will have their data recorded in one row within SPSS.

A video listed at the end of this chapter gives detailed instructions on using SPSS to carry out the McNemar test.

12.8 Describing the Effect Size

It is best to report the ratio between the total numbers who admit use in a questionnaire ($43 + 112 = 155$) to the total who do so in an interview ($6 + 112 = 118$), giving a ratio of 1.31. That suggests that a questionnaire will uncover approximately a one third greater use of cannabis than would be revealed during an interview.

12.9 How to Report the Test

12.9.1 Methods Section

In this section, you should set out the following:

- Assuming that your sample size was pre-planned, describe how this was done.
- The categorical characteristic recorded under the two different circumstances.
- The name of the statistical procedure employed (use the exact same wording as that in the menu structure of the package you used).
- Any options selected that differ from the program's defaults.
- The P-value that would be considered statistically significant.
- The name of your statistical package along with its version number and supplier.

Suitable wording might be:

A minimum sample size of 193 was determined using a spreadsheet described by Mackridge and Rowe (2018), based on a prediction that 2% of respondents would disclose cannabis use in the interview but not in the questionnaire, whilst 10% would disclose in the question-naire but not in interview. An a priori P value of <0.05 and a power of 90% power was used.

Testing was carried out using SPSS (Version 23; IBM Corporation), using the Crosstabs routine with the addition of a McNemar test.

12.9.2 Results Section

In this section, you should set out the following:

- A table arranged as in Table 12.2.
- The P-value achieved.
- Whether statistical significance was achieved.
- The total number or proportion showing one particular outcome (in the current case, admitting drug use) under one set of circumstances and the total with the same outcome under the other circumstances. If statistically significant, then quote the ratio between the two outcomes.

Suitable wording might be:

The numbers of individuals showing the various patterns of responses are shown in Table 12.2. Respondents displayed a statistically significant (P < 0.001) tendency towards greater disclosure of cannabis use in a questionnaire (32.7%) rather than in an interview (24.9%), giving a ratio of 1.31.

12.9.3 Discussion Section

A key part of your discussion will be to compare any effect size seen in your work against the minimum clinically/practically relevant difference. You will need to provide and justify a value for the latter.

This test does not generate any easily usable confidence interval for effect size. However, there are a number of options for discussing effect size and significance:

- For a non-significant result: If sample sizes are small, be wary of saying there is no effect; one may be present but you have failed to detect it. Where your sample has exceeded your calculated required sample size, you can more safely say that there is either no effect or, at the very least, any effect is very small (less than the minimum your set out in your sample size calculation) and therefore unlikely to be of any practical relevance.

- For a significant result: Discuss whether the effect size is great enough to be of practical consequence and its implications for public policy or professional practice.

12.10   Relevant Videos etc.

The following are available at
www.wiley.com/go/Mackridge/APracticalApproachtoUsingStatisticsin
HealthResearch

Videos

Video_1.1_SPSS_Basics: The absolute basics of using SPSS
Video_12.1_McNemar: Using a spreadsheet to calculate necessary sample size for a McNemar test and how to perform the test using SPSS

SPSS data files

SPSS_12.1_CannabisUse: The data for the example used to illustrate this chapter.

Spreadsheets

Spreadsheet_12.1_CannabisUse: The data for the example used to illustrate this chapter.
Spreadsheet_12.2_McNemarSampSize: Spreadsheet to calculate necessary sample size for a McNemar's test.

13

Paired T-Test

13.1   When Is the Test Applied?

Figure 13.1 shows the circumstances where a paired t-test is used:

- The factor is categorical and there are **two** different conditions.
- The outcome is a continuously varying measurement.
- All participants provide outcome results under **both** study conditions.
- Alternatively, the test can be used with matched pairs of individuals, who each provide an outcome under one of the conditions (see the final example in Table 13.1).

Note that the test only uses each individual's change in the measured outcome. In Figure 13.1, all individuals show greater values for the endpoint under the second condition. The question is whether there is convincing evidence of an overall trend toward change in one direction?

Although it might appear that the independent samples t-test could perfectly well be used in this situation, the paired test can be much more powerful and should always be used when the data is related (paired).

For full details, see Rowe (2015) chapter 13.[1]

Some examples of where the test is appropriate are shown in Table 13.1.

---

[1] Rowe P. Essential statistics for the pharmaceutical sciences, 2nd edn. Chichester: Wiley, 2015.

A Practical Approach to Using Statistics in Health Research: From Planning to Reporting, First Edition. Adam Mackridge and Philip Rowe.
© 2018 John Wiley & Sons, Inc. Published 2018 by John Wiley & Sons, Inc.
Companion website: www.wiley.com/go/Mackridge/
APracticalApproachtoUsingStatisticsinHealthResearch

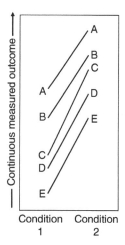

Figure 13.1 Structure of a study where a paired t-test would be used.

Table 13.1 Examples of studies that would be analyzed by a paired t-test.

Comparison made	Outcome	Question
Pre- versus post-use of a diet.	Body weight (kg)	Does the diet cause a change in weight?
One week and two weeks after moving from sea level to a high altitude residence.	Peripheral oxygen saturation	Is there further acclimatization after the first week?
Teeth dentally cleaned to remove all plaque then measure dental plaque after one month's use of a manual toothbrush. Same participant repeats whole procedure but using electric toothbrush.	Index of dental plaque	Is there any difference between the effectiveness of manual and electric toothbrushes?
Before versus after a cycle of use of a combined oral contraceptive	Systolic blood pressure	Is use of the oral contraceptive associated with any change in blood pressure?
Pairs of participants matched for sex, age, weight, and serum cholesterol prior to study. Within each pair, one will substitute an allegedly cholesterol lowering spread for butter or margarine for a three month period, while the other participant makes no change.	Change in serum cholesterol between beginning and end of study period	Does the experimental spread influence serum cholesterol levels?

13.2   An Example

For our example, we take the penultimate case in Table 13.1. Does starting to use a combined oral contraceptive (OC) lead to any change in systolic blood pressure? Participants take the OC for 28 days. Their systolic blood pressures are measured before and after the month's use. The dataset is available as an MS Excel spreadsheet or SPSS data file listed at the end of this chapter.

13.3   Presenting the Data

13.3.1   Numerically

You should report the sample size (n = 21) and the mean and standard deviation for the endpoint under both study conditions (119.5 ± 10.7 and 124.5 ± 13.7 mmHg prior to and after OC use, respectively). Additionally, you should also report the mean and SD for the changes that occurred within each individual between the two conditions (Increase of 5.0 ± 5.7 mmHg).

13.3.2   Graphically

The key values to present are the changes seen in each individual participant/institution. You could use a histogram or dot plot. Histograms require relatively large amounts of data to work effectively and dot plots may be the only effective way to represent small data sets. In the current case, there is inadequate data for a meaningful histogram, so we have produced a dot plot (Figure 13.2), which illustrates the main outcome of the experiment; there are noticeably greater numbers of positive than negative changes, suggesting that this OC does increase systolic blood pressure.

Another potential way to present the data in order to show any general trend in the measured outcome is as in Figure 13.3, which may be referred to as a "Ladder plot." This type of diagram loses its clarity if there are too many participants. In this case, it gives a good impression of the general upward trend in blood pressure.

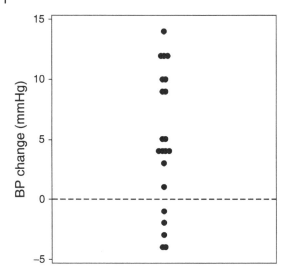

Figure 13.2 Dot plot showing changes in systolic blood pressure (mmHg) after one month's use of a combined oral contraceptive.

13.4 Data Requirements

13.4.1 Variables Required

You will require two continuously measured variables (columns in SPSS) that describe the same measured outcome under the two conditions. Each row represents the pair of values from one participant or matched pair of participants.

13.4.2 Normal Distribution of the Outcome Data

It is not a requirement that the two sets of outcome values (in the current case, the pre- and post-treatment blood pressures) are normally distributed. However, it is a requirement that the individual changes in outcome between the two conditions are approximately normally distributed, as this is the data that the statistical test will be examining.

Section 2.2.1 describes how to test for normality. This is a relatively small data set and detection of non-normality is not easy. However, Figure 13.2 shows no evidence of the data breaking up into distinct clusters (polymodality) nor is there any sign of skewness: i.e. we do

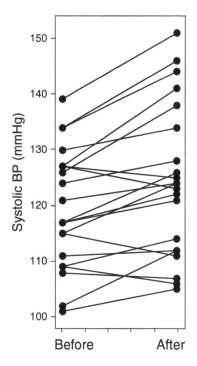

Figure 13.3 A ladder plot of systolic blood pressures (mmHg) before and after one month's use of a combined oral contraceptive.

not see a high proportion of the data points clustered at either the low or high end of the range of observed values. We have also produced a normal probability plot (Figure 13.4) to check for long tails in our data, and everything looks good here. See a video listed at the end of this chapter for details of using statistical packages to check for normality.

As neither Figures 13.2 nor 13.4 give cause for concern, it is reasonable to treat the blood pressure changes as being normally distributed.

If the individual changes do not form a normal distribution and the problem is positive skew, it may be possible to convert the data to normality using the log transform (see video listed at end of the chapter). If the data cannot be successfully transformed, then you can instead use the non-parametric Wilcoxon signed rank test (see Chapter 14).

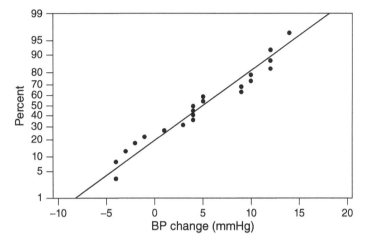

Figure 13.4 Normal probability plot of the individual changes in systolic blood pressure used to test for any evidence of a long-tailed distribution.

13.4.3   Equal Standard Deviations

The paired t-test only uses one set of values (the individual changes in outcome), so there is no issue of equal SDs

13.4.4   Equal Sample Sizes

There must obviously be equal numbers of data points in the two initial data sets. Unfortunately, if one value has been lost for a particular individual or matched pair, the other value will have to be discarded, as no individual change can be calculated for that individual/pair.

13.5   An Outline of the Test

Three aspects of the data will determine whether your results are statistically significant:

- How far the mean value among the individual changes diverges from zero: A mean value near zero is less likely to be significant than one well away from zero.
- The size of your sample: the larger your sample, The greater the chances of statistical significance.

- The standard deviation among the individual changes: Highly varying values are less likely to be statistically significant than consistent ones.

13.6 Planning Sample Sizes

To calculate necessary sample size, you will need four values:

- The smallest mean change that you consider to be practically/clinically meaningful. The closer to zero this value is, the larger the sample size you will need (big differences can be detected by small samples).
- The anticipated standard deviation among the individual changes. Section 6.2 discusses the problem of trying to anticipate the SD for your data prior to collection.
- The power you require – see glossary. Higher powers (90% or 95%) require larger sample sizes. A figure of 90% is commonly used, but where data is difficult to obtain, this could be reduced to 80%.
- What P-value[2] will be considered as statistically significant. A value of less than 0.05 is usually appropriate.

See a video listed at the end of this chapter for detailed instructions on using G*Power to calculate a sample size.

13.7 Carrying Out the Test

See a video listed at the end of this chapter for detailed instructions on using SPSS to carry out the paired t-test.

13.8 Describing the Effect Size

The effect size will be described as the mean among the individual changes in outcome between the two conditions and its 95% confidence interval.

---

[2] This may be referred to in software packages as "Alpha" – see glossary.

13.9   How to Report the Test

13.9.1   Methods Section

In this section, you should set out the following:

- How your sample size was calculated (If it was not pre-calculated, say why not; maybe all available cases in a pre-existing database were used.)
- The continuously varying measured parameter used to record the endpoint under the two conditions.
- The name of the statistical analysis employed (use the exact same wording as that in the menu structure of the package you used).
- Any options selected.
- The P-value that would be considered as statistically significant.
- The name of your statistical package along with its version number and supplier.

Suitable wording might be:

> The minimum sample size was calculated to be 20, based on a minimum clinically meaningful change in BP of 5mmHg and an estimated standard deviation among the changes in BP of 7.5 mmHg (*give references or justification*). An a priori value of P was set at <0.05, and a power of 80% was used in the calculation, which was carried out using G*Power (Version 3.1; Heinrich-Heine-Universität, Düsseldorf).
>
> The "Paired-Samples T-Test" routine in SPSS (Version 23; IBM Corporation) was used to carry out the main analysis.

13.9.2   Results Section

In this section, you should set out the following:

- The valid sample size (excluding any data where only one of the two values are available).
- A statement concerning normal distribution in the data.
- The mean and SD for the endpoint in both data sets.
- A histogram or dot plot of the individual changes or a ladder plot of the two sets of results; the choice will depend to an extent upon your sample sizes – figures similar to Figure 13.2 or 13.3.

- The P-value and a statement as to whether statistical significance was achieved.
- The mean among the individual changes and its 95% confidence interval.

Suitable wording might be:

> A total of 21 participants completed the study, with mean (± SD) systolic blood pressure before and after use of the oral contraceptive being 119.5 ± 10.7 and 124.5 ± 13.7 mmHg respectively. Individual changes in blood pressure are shown in Figure 13.2; this, along with a normal probability plot, showed no marked deviation from normal distribution. There was a statistically significant (P=0.001) increase in systolic blood pressure of 5.0 ± 5.7 (95% CI 2.4 to 7.5) mmHg following one month's use of the oral contraceptive.

13.9.3 Discussion Section

It would be appropriate to explore the following points relating to your statistical analysis. Within this, you will need to provide and justify a value for the clinically/practically relevant difference.

- See Sections 6.5 and 6.6 for guidance on interpreting statistically significant or non-significant results.
- Whether or not statistically significant – the implications for public policy or professional practice.

13.10   Relevant Videos etc.

The following are available at www.wiley.com/go/Mackridge/APracticalApproachtoUsingStatisticsin HealthResearch

Videos

Video_1.1_SPSS_Basics: The absolute basics of using SPSS

Video_2.1_Normality testing: Using SPSS to determine whether measured data follows a normal distribution and log transformation to improve normality

Video_13.1_Paired_t_SampSize: Using G*Power for paired t sample size calculation

Video_13.2_Paired_t: Using SPSS to perform a paired t-test

SPSS data files

SPSS_13.1_OralContracep: The data for the example used to illustrate this chapter.

Spreadsheets

Spreadsheet_13.1_OralContracep: The data for the example used to illustrate this chapter.

14

Wilcoxon Signed Rank Test

This test is also known as the Wilcoxon paired samples test.

14.1   When Is the Test Applied?

Figure 14.1 shows the circumstances where a Wilcoxon signed rank test is used:

- The factor is categorical with **two** different conditions or time points.
- The outcome is an ordinal variable (or a continuously varying measured variable where the changes that occur are not normally distributed).
- All participants provide outcome results under **both** study conditions.
- Alternatively, the test can be used with matched pairs of individuals, who each provide an outcome under one of the conditions (see the final example in Table 14.1).

Note that the test only uses the changes in the ordinal endpoint; the fact that individual A produces higher values in both conditions than J is irrelevant. In the figure, all individuals show equal or lower values for the endpoint under the second condition, with no increases. The question is whether there is convincing evidence of an overall downward trend in outcome values for Condition 2 compared to Condition 1.

For full details, see Rowe (2015)[1] section 21.4.1.

---

[1] Rowe P. Essential statistics for the pharmaceutical sciences, 2nd edn. Chichester: Wiley, 2015.

A Practical Approach to Using Statistics in Health Research: From Planning to Reporting, First Edition. Adam Mackridge and Philip Rowe.
© 2018 John Wiley & Sons, Inc. Published 2018 by John Wiley & Sons, Inc.
Companion website: www.wiley.com/go/Mackridge/
APracticalApproachtoUsingStatisticsinHealthResearch

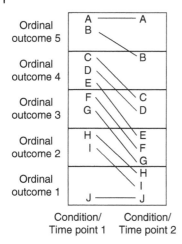

Figure 14.1 Structure of a study where a Wilcoxon signed rank test would be used.

Some examples where this test would be used are shown in Table 14.1.

14.2   An Example

In our example, we take the first case in Table 14.1. Is a new system for booking clinic appointments perceived as better/worse than the original system? The dataset is available as an SPSS data file and an MS Excel spreadsheet as listed at the end of this chapter.

14.3   Presenting the Data

14.3.1   Numerically

You could use a table such as Table 14.2 to report the numbers of individuals who select each of the available levels of outcome at the two stages of the study.

The median for five-point scales is notoriously insensitive and it may sometimes be appropriate to use the mean and SD (see Appendix 1 in Chapter 3). However, for the current data set, the median satisfaction

Table 14.1 Examples of studies that would be analyzed by a Wilcoxon signed rank test.

Comparison made	Outcome	Question
Patients' opinions concerning a clinic's appointments booking system gathered before and after the implementation of a new system.	Satisfaction scale (1=Very dissatisfied; 2 = Dissatisfied; 3 = Neutral; 4 = Satisfied; 5 = Very satisfied). Each patient provided a grading both before and after the change.	Was the new system viewed as more/less satisfactory than the old one?
Patients with chronic lower back pain assessed before and after training in Pilates.	Self-assessed score from disability questionnaire (Score range 0 – 11).	Is Pilates training followed by a change in perceived disability?
Children attending a school near a main road that is to be pedestrianized. Each child is studied before and after closure of the road.	Percentage of hemoglobin present as carboxy-haemoglobin (a marker of carbon monoxide exposure). Individual changes are markedly non-normal and cannot be satisfactorily transformed to normality.	Is there any change in carbon monoxide exposure following road closure?
Pairs of dental technicians matched for gender, age, and years of employment. Within each pair, one had been on at least one training course during the previous year and the other had not.	Score on a five-point scale for their sense of being a valued part of their professional team (Ranging from "Very strong" to "Not at all").	Is attendance at a training scheme associated with a higher/lower sense of being professionally valued?

score was four before and three after the change in the system, indicating that there was a decline in satisfaction, and the median will suffice in this case.

However, as this is a paired study, it is often helpful to describe the pattern of changes in the opinions of individual participants (satisfaction after the change minus satisfaction before). You could then report the median and inter-quartile range (IQR) among these changes (Median = −1, IQR = 1).

Table 14.2 Numbers of individuals expressing various levels of satisfaction with an appointment booking system, before and after change to system. Higher scores represent greater levels of satisfaction.

Satisfaction score	Old system	New system
1 (very dissatisfied)	11	17
2 (dissatisfied)	7	24
3 (neutral)	21	26
4 (satisfied)	42	25
5 (very satisfied)	23	12

Finally, you might decide that the target is a response of Satisfied or Very satisfied and hence report that 65 (63%) indicated satisfaction before the change, but this fell to 37 (36%) afterwards.

14.3.2 Graphically

You could use bar charts to show either the pattern of outcome scores under both study conditions or alternatively, to show the individual changes in scores. Figure 14.2 shows the satisfaction scores before and after the change to the booking system: high levels of satisfaction are less frequent after the change. An alternative approach is shown in Figure 14.3, which shows the individual changes in satisfaction; the preponderance of negative over positive changes is fairly obvious.

14.4   Data Requirements

14.4.1   Variables Required

You will require two variables (columns in SPSS) which describe the outcome data under the two conditions. Each row represents the pair of values from one participant or matched pair of participants. For our example, we would need one for satisfaction before and one for after the introduction of the new system. (In SPSS, you will have to declare the outcome as Scale even if it is actually ordinal. Otherwise the test will not be calculated.)

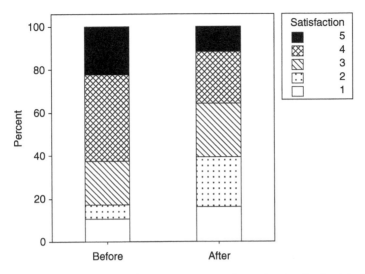

Figure 14.2 Proportions of participants expressing various levels of satisfaction with the appointment booking system before and after introduction of the new system. Higher scores represent higher levels of satisfaction.

14.4.2 Normal Distributions and Equal Standard Deviations

The test is non-parametric so there are no requirements for normality or equal standard deviations.

14.4.3 Equal Sample Sizes

There must be equal numbers of observations under the two conditions. If, for any individual, you do not have data under one of the conditions, then that participant has to be removed from the analysis.

14.5 An Outline of the Test

The outcome depends upon the degree of imbalance between positive and negative individual changes (as in Figure 14.3). If it is clear that positive changes are more numerous and/or of greater magnitude

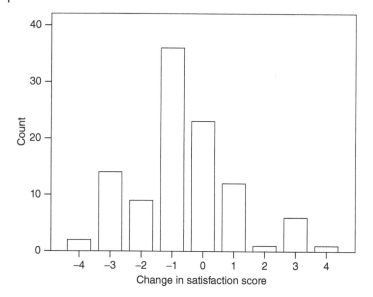

Figure 14.3 Bar chart of individual changes in satisfaction scores following introduction of the new appointment booking system. Negative and positive figures represent reduced or increased satisfaction, respectively.

than negative changes (or vice versa), significance is likely. As with all tests, the larger the sample size, the greater the chances of statistical significance.

14.6   Planning Sample Sizes

An exact calculation of necessary sample sizes for a study to be analyzed by a Wilcoxon signed rank test is not straightforward. However, a pragmatic approach can be based upon the fact that even with the most unfavorable circumstances, the power of a Wilcoxon signed rank test is 86% of that achieved by applying a paired t-test to the same data. Taking this approach, you can follow the procedure to calculate sample sizes required for a paired t-test and then **add** 15%. This will give adequate sample sizes when you apply a Wilcoxon signed rank test to the results.

See Chapter 13 and the video listed at the end of this chapter for detailed instructions on using G*Power to calculate sample sizes for a paired t-test.

14.7 Carrying Out the Test

See the video listed at the end of this chapter for detailed instructions on using SPSS to carry out the Wilcoxon signed rank test.

14.8 Describing the Effect Size

There are several possible approaches to describing the extent of the difference between the two situations, and no single one is applicable in all cases. You should review the discussion in Section 14.3 and consider what is appropriate for your particular study. The main options are:

- Report the difference between the median values for the two data sets. This may be a very insensitive indicator of difference and can be zero, i.e. equal medians for the two groups despite the test indicating a statistically significant difference.
- If the medians fail to illustrate the difference, report the difference between the mean values for the two groups. This should be an addition to, not a substitute for, reporting the medians. Explain why it was necessary to use the means owing to the insensitivity of the median in relation to your data.
- Report the median and/or mean among the individual differences in the outcome variable when comparing the two study conditions.
- Contrast the proportion of scores above/below a critical level in the two sets of data. This is most likely to be appropriate where there would be broad agreement that scores above a certain value are satisfactory while those below are unsatisfactory (or vice versa). As an example, AUDIT (Alcohol Use Disorders Identification Test) scores of sixteen or more would generally be accepted as indicating a high enough risk associated with the pattern of alcohol use to justify referral to a specialist service.

14.9 How to Report the Test

14.9.1 Methods Section

In this section, you should set out the following:

- How your sample size was calculated (if it was not pre-calculated, say why not).
- The variable used to record the ordinal or continuous measured outcome under the two conditions.
- The name of the statistical analysis employed (use the exact same wording as that in the menu structure of the package you used).
- Any options selected if these differ from the program's defaults.
- The P-value that would be considered as statistically significant.
- The name of your statistical package along with its version number and supplier.

Suitable wording might be:

> A minimum sample size of 97 was calculated using the approach described in Mackridge and Rowe (2018), based on the minimum meaningful difference being a change of 0.5 in the opinion score (*give references or justification*) and that the standard deviation among these changes would be 1.5 points (*references or justification*). An a priori value of P was set at <0.05 to indicate significance and 90% power was required.
>
> The satisfaction scores under the two conditions were compared via the non-parametric related samples procedure in SPSS (Version 23; IBM Corporation).

14.9.2 Results Section

In this section, you should set out the following:

- The number of participants.
- The observed outcomes described by any of the methods set out in Section 14.3.
- A measure of effect size using any of the suggestions in Section 14.8.
- If the original data was continuous measured, describe its distribution and state why a non-parametric test was used.
- The P-value for the test and a statement as to whether the result is statistically significant.

Suitable wording might be

A total of 104 participants provided valid responses for both time points. Figure 14.3 shows the frequencies for the various positive and negative changes in individuals' responses on the satisfaction scale. There was a statistically significant (P < 0.001) reduction in satisfaction following the introduction of the new booking system, with those describing themselves as Satisfied or Very satisfied falling from 65 (63%) prior to the change to 37 (36%) afterwards.

14.9.3   Discussion Section

A key part of your discussion will be to compare the effect size seen in your work against the minimum clinically/practically relevant difference. You will need to provide and justify a value for the latter.

Non-parametric methods do not generate any easily usable confidence interval for effect size. However, there are a number of options for discussing effect size and significance:

- For a non-significant result: If sample sizes are small, be wary of saying there is no effect; one may be present but you have failed to detect it. Where your sample has exceeded your calculated required sample size, and the variance (SD) is no larger than that used in your calculation, you can more safely say that there is either no effect or, at the very least, any effect is very small (less than the minimum you set out in your sample size calculation) and therefore unlikely to be of any practical relevance.
- For a significant result: Discuss whether the effect size is great enough to be of practical consequence and its implications for public policy or professional practice.

14.10   Relevant Videos etc.

The following are available at
www.wiley.com/go/Mackridge/APracticalApproachtoUsingStatisticsin HealthResearch

Videos

Video_1.1_SPSS_Basics: The absolute basics of using SPSS

Video_13.1_Paired_t_SampSize: Using G*Power for paired t sample size calculation

Video_14.1_WilcoxonSignedRank: Using SPSS to carry out a Wilcoxon signed rank test

SPSS data files

SPSS_14.1_AppointmentBooking. The data used to illustrate this chapter.

Spreadsheets

Spreadheet_14.1_AppointmentBooking.xlsx. The data used to illustrate this chapter.

15

Repeated Measures Analysis of Variance

15.1 When Is the Test Applied?

Figure 15.1 shows the circumstances where a repeated measures Analysis of Variance (ANOVA) is used:

- The factor is categorical and there are **three** or more different times or study conditions.
- The outcome is a continuously varying measurement.
- All participants provide outcome results under **all** study conditions.

Note that the test only takes account of the changes that occur within each individual participant. The fact that participant A produces consistently higher values than E is irrelevant. What is being tested is the apparent trend, across all participants, for their values to be high under condition 3 and low under condition 2.

This test is well suited to longitudinal studies that track an outcome over time. A common scenario for this test is where participants are studied prior to and shortly after an intervention such as a training program, to see if a change occurs, but they are then studied again after a longer period to see if the intervention produced a lasting effect.

In principle, the model allows any number times/conditions to be studied, but it can become very difficult to interpret the results if too many variants are considered. As ever, our advice is "keep it simple" and limit yourself to the minimum useful number of conditions/time-points.

A Practical Approach to Using Statistics in Health Research: From Planning to Reporting, First Edition. Adam Mackridge and Philip Rowe.
© 2018 John Wiley & Sons, Inc. Published 2018 by John Wiley & Sons, Inc.
Companion website: www.wiley.com/go/Mackridge/
APracticalApproachtoUsingStatisticsinHealthResearch

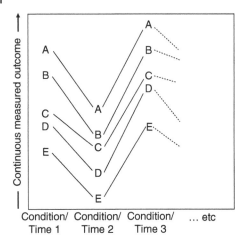

Figure 15.1 Structure of a study where a repeated measures analysis of variance would be used.

Whenever a repeated measures ANOVA is applicable, it would be possible to use the simple one-way analysis of variance. However, the repeated measures test is more powerful and is therefore preferable.

Some examples of where this test would be used are shown in Table 15.1.

15.2   An Example

For our example, we take the first case in Table 15.1: Does dietary training lead to short/longer term weight changes? A dataset for 106 participants is available as an MS Excel spreadsheet or SPSS data file listed at the end of this chapter.

15.3   Presenting the Data

Table 15.2 contains part of the data (the first ten participants) from our diet example. This will be used to illustrate a number of general points. The first three columns give the weights of participants at the three time points, and the fourth column gives each individual patient's change in weight between the baseline and one month time points. The next column gives the differences in weight between the

Table 15.1 Examples of studies that would be analyzed by a repeated measures analysis of variance.

Comparison made	Outcome	Question
Prior to, three months after, and one year after training in the use of a weight reducing diet.	Body weight (kg)	Does the diet cause a short term and/or sustained change in weight?
Prior to the use of Oral Contraceptives (OC), at the end of a cycle of use of a progestogen only OC, and then at the end of a cycle of use of a combined OC.	Systolic blood pressure	Is use of either or both of the types of oral contra-ceptives associated with any change in blood pressure?
Patients with chronic lower back pain, at baseline, one month after and six months after exercise training.	Visual analog pain scale (Scores cover a range of 0–100)	Does the training cause short and/or long-term changes in pain levels?

three month and one year time points, and finally we have the differences between the beginning and end of the study.

15.3.1 Numerical Presentation of the Data

Assuming space permits, it would be ideal to show the mean and standard deviation for the endpoint at each stage of the study conditions (i.e. a summary of the data in the first three columns of Table 15.2) and also the means and SDs among the individual changes that occur (i.e. a summary of the data in the final three columns of Table 15.2). If this is not possible, you will have to decide which information is most important in the context of your study. For the current example, the most important information is probably the mean and SD among the individual responses to the diet, however it would also be important for the reader to know the mean weight prior to dieting, as this indicates the extent of obesity among the participants.

15.3.2 Graphical Presentation of the Data

With small numbers of participants, it may be possible to use a ladder plot (as shown in Figure 15.2; first ten participants only). These are quite informative as they allow the reader to track individuals as they

Table 15.2 Weights of participants (kg) at the three time points, and the differences in weight comparing all possible pairs of time points (first ten participants only). Each row represents one participant.

	Weight: Baseline	Weight: Three month	Weight: One year	Difference: Baseline and Three month	Difference: Three month and One year	Difference: Baseline and One year
	127	107	100	−20	−7	−27
	105	89	86	−16	−3	−19
	132	116	125	−16	9	−7
	121	106	108	−15	2	−13
	106	90	98	−16	8	−8
	118	108	112	−10	4	−6
	123	111	111	−12	0	−12
	112	99	108	−13	9	−4
	105	91	101	−14	10	−4
	116	96	90	−20	−6	−26
Mean	116.5	101.3	105.9	−15.2	4.6	−10.6
SD	9.5	9.6	3.3	1.0	1.4	1.8

progress through the various stages of the study, but they become impossibly complicated even with only moderate sample sizes; if too many lines are plotted, it is no longer possible to follow any of them. Figure 15.2 clearly shows an initial drop in weight and a partial rebound in weight at one year. If the number of participants is too great for a ladder plot, then you could produce a plot of the mean (±SD) for the outcome at each stage of the study as in Figure 15.3, which summarizes the results for the full data set. This also shows a fall and rebound in weights.

15.4 Data Requirements

15.4.1 Variables Required

You will require a variable (column in SPSS) which describe the outcome data for each of the conditions/time-points. Each row represents the values from one participant. For our example, we

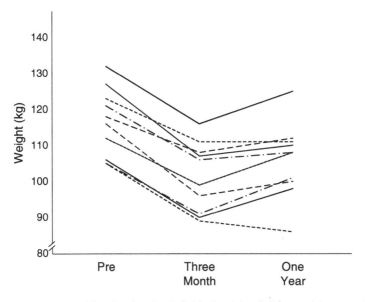

Figure 15.2 Ladder plot showing individual weights (kg) for participants at the three time points in the study (first ten individuals only).

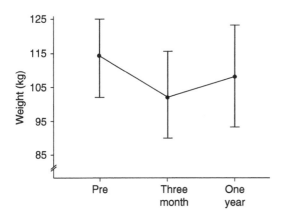

Figure 15.3 Weights (kg) of participants at the three time points in the study (mean ± SD). (Data for all 106 participants are described.)

would need three columns, for the baseline, three month follow-up, and one year follow-up.

15.4.2 Normal Distribution of the Outcome Data

There is no requirement for a normal distribution among the outcome values for each condition/time point (the first three columns of Table 15.2). However, there is a requirement that the changes that occur as individuals progress from one stage of the study to another (final three columns of Table 15.2) are approximately normally distributed. A video listed at the end of this chapter will show you how to check for normal distribution. If it emerges that there is a severe problem of non-normality, you should instead use the non-parametric Friedman's test (Chapter 16).

15.4.3 Equal Standard Deviations

As in the previous section, the differences in weights between time points are what concern us (the final three columns in Table 15.2), and these should display approximate equality among their SDs (See Section 6.1).

15.4.4 Equal Sample Sizes

There must be equal numbers of data points for all the conditions/ time points studied – If one value has been lost for a particular individual, the other data points for that individual cannot be included in the analysis. If there is a lot of missing data, you should consider the appropriateness of carrying out this test; you could instead use a one-way analysis of variance (Chapter 10). While the one-way test is less powerful than the repeated measures version, it could use all the data, which might outweigh the power difference.

15.5   An Outline of the Test

Three aspects of the data will determine whether your results are statistically significant:

- How far the mean values for the individual changes shown in the final three columns of Table 15.2 diverge from zero. If any of these mean values are clearly above or below zero, this indicates a major difference between two of the study conditions, and it is then likely that statistical significance will be achieved.

- The size of your samples: it is very difficult for small samples to provide adequate evidence of any real differences, whereas large samples are more likely to be statistically significant.
- The standard deviations among the individual changes in the final three columns of Table 15.2: highly varying values will make statistical significance less likely.

15.6   Planning Sample Sizes

An exact calculation of necessary sample size for a repeated measures ANOVA is complex and probably too challenging for a reader of this introductory text. Do not be put off undertaking a research project just because of this stage in the process. If you already have data, simply analyze all that is available. If you need to collect new data, it is often reasonable to allow practicality to drive your sample size (i.e. the number of cases for which you can collect data within the resources and time available). This would be unlikely to be sufficient for a large funding body, but when submitting grants to a major funder, we would recommend including a statistician in the planning process for your study, as planning such large-scale, complex studies goes beyond the scope of this book.

It is possible to guage an approximate sample size. The key point is the relationship between the mean and variability of the numbers in the last three columns of Table 15.2. You first need to identify which pair of conditions are expected to show the greatest contrast. In our example, we might decide that this would be between the baseline weight and that after three months. You then need to estimate the mean and SD for the relevant contrast (in our case, this would equate to the mean and SD for the figures in the fourth column of Table 15.2). Finally, calculate the ratio of the mean to the SD. Table 15.3 then indicates appropriate sample sizes. If, for example, you think that the mean and SD among the differences are likely to be similar in size (a ratio of 1.0), then a sample size of 25 should suffice. If you have no idea what the mean and/or SD of the differences are likely to be, you may need to start with a pilot experiment to estimate these figures and then finalize a plan. See section 6.2 for further discussion on estimating sample sizes.

Table 15.3 Appropriate sample sizes for a repeated measures analysis of variance.

Mean divided by SD	Sample size
0.50	75
0.75	40
1.00	25
1.25	20
1.50	15

Table 15.3 assumes that there are three study conditions or time points. For more complex designs, somewhat greater sample sizes will be required, but these fall beyond the scope of this book.

15.7 Carrying Out the Test

See a video listed at the end of this chapter for detailed instructions on using SPSS to carry out a repeated measures ANOVA.

15.8 Describing the Effect Size

The effect size would be described as the mean differences (with confidence intervals) between the various stages or conditions. In the current case, you would almost certainly want to report the mean reduction in weight from baseline to the three month point and the change from baseline up to one year, as estimates of the short term and sustained effect of the diet. If space permits, reporting the mean increase between three months and a year would also be useful.

It is likely that you will report several mean differences between time points, each with its own confidence interval, which means you should be aware of multiplicity (See Chapter 5). Steps need to be taken to avoid inflating the risk that one of your confidence intervals may not include the true value and so the accompanying video (see end of chapter) includes the use of the Bonferroni correction.

15.9   How to Report the Test

15.9.1   Methods Section

In this section, you should set out the following:

- Sample size calculation – how was this done, or if not pre-calculated, how was it estimated/what were the driving criteria?
- The continuously varying measurement used to record the endpoint for the various different times/conditions.
- The name of the statistical analysis employed. Refer to it as a "Repeated measures analysis of variance."
- Any options selected that differ from the program's defaults.
- The P-value that would be considered as statistically significant.
- The name of your statistical package along with its version number and supplier.

Suitable wording might be:

> A minimum sample size of 75 was selected based on the method described by Mackridge and Rowe (2018) (*give this book as a reference*). It was anticipated that the greatest contrast would be between weights prior to dieting and those at the three-month time point. The predicted mean weight change over this period was 5 kg, with a standard deviation of 10 kg. The main analysis was by a repeated measures analysis of variance implemented as a General Linear Model (Repeated Measures) using SPSS (Version 23; IBM Corporation). The test would be considered statistically significant if the P-value was less than 0.05. For follow-up comparisons between pairs of time points, the Bonferroni correction was applied.

15.9.2   Results Section

There are a number of ways to present this data. These include graphs such as Figures 15.2 and 15.3 or a table as in Table 15.4. You will need to consider which information is most important in the context of your study and also how much information your word-count will allow. In the current case you might provide:

- The sample size.
- The mean and standard deviation for the endpoint at the beginning of the study.

Table 15.4 Changes in weight (kg) when comparing various pairs of time points. Means, SDs and 95% confidence intervals (Bonferroni corrected) are shown.

Comparison made	Baseline versus Three months	Three months versus One year	Baseline versus One year
Mean ± SD	−11.0 ±8.3	+4.6 ±8.7	−6.4 ±11.7
95% CI	−9.0 to −12.9	+2.5 to +6.6	−3.6 to −9.1

- A graph similar to Figure 15.3.
- The mean and SD for individual differences in the endpoint when comparing pairs of time points (Bonferroni corrected confidence intervals should be added).
- The P-value for the overall test of statistical significance.
- A statement as to whether overall statistical significance was achieved and also whether each of the contrasts between pairs of time points were statistically significant.

Suitable wording might be:

> The number of participants completing the study was 106. Mean weight (± SD) prior to dieting was 114.3 ± 10.9 kg. The overall analysis of variance was statistically significant ($P < 0.001$). The mean changes in individuals' weights between various pairs of time points are shown in Table 15.4 along with SDs and 95% confidence intervals (Bonferroni corrected). The data demonstrates that, compared to baseline, there was a statistically significant weight reduction at three months, which was sustained, albeit with a moderate rebound, at one year.

15.9.3 Discussion Section

It would be appropriate to explore the following points relating to your statistical analysis. Within this, you will need to provide and justify a value for the clinically/practically relevant difference.

- See Sections 6.5 and 6.6 for guidance on interpreting statistically significant or non-significant results.
- Whether or not statistically significant – the implications for public policy or professional practice.

15.10   Relevant Videos etc.

The following are available at
www.wiley.com/go/Mackridge/APracticalApproachtoUsingStatisticsin
HealthResearch

Videos

Video_1.1_SPSS_Basics: The absolute basics of using SPSS
Video_2.1_Normality testing: Using SPSS to determine whether measured data follows a normal distribution and log transformation to improve normality
Video_15_1_RepMeasures: Using SPSS to perform a repeated measures analysis of variance and Bonferroni corrected follow-up tests

SPSS data files

SPSS_15.1_DietWeights: The data for the example used to illustrate this chapter.

Spreadsheets

Spreadsheet_15.1_DietWeights: The data for the example used to illustrate this chapter.

16

Friedman Test

16.1 When Is the Test Applied?

Figure 16.1 shows the circumstances where a Friedman test is used:

- The factor is categorical with **three** or more different times or study conditions.
- The outcome is an ordinal variable (or a continuously varying measured variable where the individual changes that occur are not normally distributed).
- All participants provide outcome results under **all** study conditions.

Note that the test only takes account of the changes that occur within each individual participant. The fact that participant A produces consistently higher scores than E is irrelevant. What is being tested is the apparent trend, across all subjects, for their scores to be low under condition 2.

A common scenario for this test is where subjects are studied prior to and shortly after an intervention (e.g. training) to see if a change occurs, but they are then studied again after a longer period to see if the intervention produced a lasting effect.

In principle, the model allows any number times/conditions to be studied, but it can become very difficult to interpret the results if too many variants are considered. As ever, our advice is "keep it simple" and limit yourself to the minimum number of useful conditions/time-points.

Some examples of where this test would be used are shown in Table 16.1.

A Practical Approach to Using Statistics in Health Research: From Planning to Reporting, First Edition. Adam Mackridge and Philip Rowe.
© 2018 John Wiley & Sons, Inc. Published 2018 by John Wiley & Sons, Inc.
Companion website: www.wiley.com/go/Mackridge/
APracticalApproachtoUsingStatisticsinHealthResearch

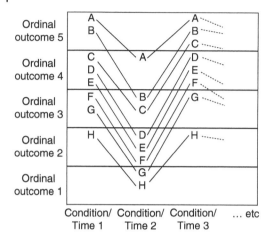

Figure 16.1 Structure of a study where a Friedman test would be used.

Table 16.1 Examples of studies that would be analyzed by a Friedman test.

Comparison made	Outcome	Question
Individual children taste each of three different liquid formulations of a medicine for children.	Acceptability of taste (Ordinal scale: 1 = Very unpleasant; 2 = Rather unpleasant 3 = OK; 4 = Quite pleasant; 5 = Very pleasant.)	Are there differences among the formulations in terms of taste acceptability?
Three advisory leaflets – old text version, new text version, and new image-based version.	Measure of clarity, using a four-point scale (Higher scores equal greater clarity), scored by individuals who each look at ALL leaflets	Are there differences in clarity between the various versions?
Children assessed before, one week after, and three months after training in tooth brushing technique.	Dental hygiene rated 1 = Poor; 2 = Fair; 3 = Good; 4 = Excellent	Does the training lead to short and/or long term changes in dental hygiene?
Prior to, three months after, and one year after training in the use of a weight reducing diet.	Body weight (kg). The data does not meet the normality requirement for a repeated measures ANOVA set out in Section 15.4.2	Does the diet cause a short term and/or sustained change in weight?

16.2 An Example

For our example, we take the third case in Table 16.1: Does tooth brushing training lead to short term and/or sustained changes in dental hygiene? A dataset for 43 participants is available as an MS Excel spreadsheet or SPSS data sheet listed at the end of this chapter.

16.3 Presenting the Data

Several possible methods for presenting the data are provided. One method may work well with one study, and in other cases, something else may be appropriate. The choice will depend upon the details of your study and its outcomes.

16.3.1 Bar Charts of the Outcomes at Various Stages

You could present the numbers recorded as having each level of dental hygiene at the three stages of the study, as in Figure 16.2. This shows the increased proportions with the higher grades (Good or Excellent) one week after training, but also their subsequent decline after three months.

Alternatively, you could show the numbers of participants who demonstrate various degrees of improvement (or deterioration) compared to their initial score, as in Figure 16.3. "Plus two" indicates an individual who has improved their score by two grades, "Minus one" is a deterioration of one grade and "Zero" is no change. (This could also be rendered as a stacked bar chart, more similar to Figure 16.2.) Positive changes are in a clear majority over negative ones at the one week stage, but by three months, the commonest outcome is no change with small and approximately equal numbers showing improvement and deterioration.

16.3.2 Summarizing the Data via Medians or Means

With an ordinal scale as narrow as that in the current case (only four points wide), medians are very insensitive and can provide only a crude reflection of the outcomes. Consequently, you may need to additionally provide the mean values. If the mean is required, you should explain the inadequacy of the median and use this as justification for

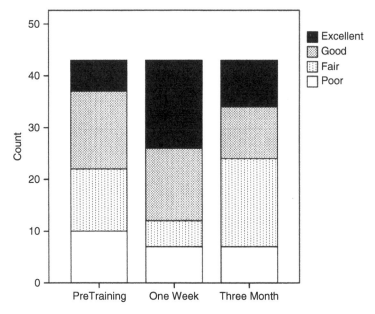

Figure 16.2 Stacked bar chart showing dental hygiene scores prior to, one week after, and three months after training in tooth brushing technique.

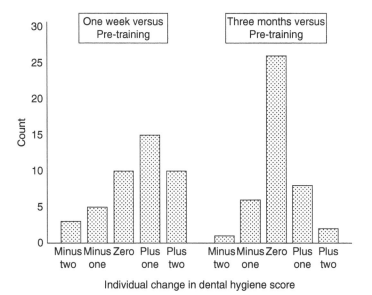

Figure 16.3 Bar chart showing individual changes in dental hygiene scores one week after and three months after training in tooth brushing technique.

Table 16.2 Descriptive statistics for dental hygiene scores prior to, one week after, and three months after training in tooth brushing technique.

Period	Median	Mean	SD
Pre-training	2	2.40	1.00
One week	3	2.95	1.09
Three months	2	2.49	1.01

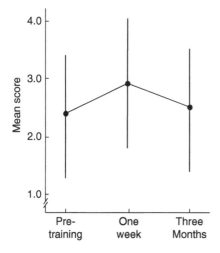

Figure 16.4 Mean dental hygiene scores (± SD) at the three time points in the study.

the addition of the means (See Section 3.2). The medians, means, and SDs for the scores at all three stages of the experiment are shown in Table 16.2 and the means and SDs in Figure 16.4.

16.3.3 Splitting the Data at Some Critical Point in the Scale

As described in Section 3.2.3, it may be clinically relevant to split the original scale at some point into two (lower and higher) ranges. In the current case, you might feel that a realistic target was either of the top two grades (Good or Excellent) and therefore report the proportions achieving this target at the pre-training, one week, and three months stages. These were 49%, 72%, and 44%, respectively. If you do this, see the warning in Section 3.2.3 about carrying out statistical analyses with the data in this format.

16.4 Data Requirements

16.4.1 Variables Required

You will require a variable (column in SPSS) that describes the outcome data for each of the conditions/time-points. Each row represents the values from one participant. For our example, we would need three columns, for the baseline, one week follow up, and three month follow up. (In SPSS, you will have to declare the outcome as Scale even if it is actually ordinal. Otherwise the test will not be calculated.)

16.4.2 Normal Distribution and Standard Deviations in the Outcome Data

This is a nonparametric test, and there is no requirement for normal distributions or equal standard deviations.

16.4.3 Equal Sample Sizes

There must be equal numbers of data points for all the conditions/ time points studied – If one value has been lost for a particular individual, the other data points for that individual cannot be included in the analysis. If there is a lot of missing data, you should consider the appropriateness of carrying out this test; you could instead use a Kruskal–Wallis test (Chapter 11). While the Kruskal–Wallis test is less powerful than Friedman's, it could use all the data, which might outweigh the power difference.

16.5 An Outline of the Test

The individual changes that occur when individuals move from one time point or study condition to another will determine whether your result is statistically significant. Figure 16.3 presents the data in a particularly relevant manner. The left hand part of the figure – the contrast between pre-training and the one week time point – shows a fairly strong imbalance, with more positive than negative changes among individuals' scores. This is likely to produce a statistically significant outcome. In contrast, in the comparison between pre-training and three months (right hand section of figure), a high proportion show no change, and positive and negative changes are roughly balanced. This would contribute very little toward statistical significance.

Overall, the test is likely to be statistically significant so long as at least one pair of the study times/conditions show a strong contrast. The lack of contrast between pre-training and three months will reduce the chances of significance, but the clear change from pre-training to the one week time point will probably suffice to guarantee significance.

16.6   Planning Sample Sizes

An exact pre-calculation of necessary sample size for a Friedman test is probably unrealistic in the context of the sort of moderate-scale, modest-budget study described as our target in Section 1.2. Do not be put off undertaking a research project just because of this stage in the process. If you already have data, simply analyze all that is available. If you need to collect new data, it is reasonable to allow practicality to drive your sample size (i.e. the number of cases for which you can collect data within the resources and time available). This would be unlikely to be sufficient for a large funding body, but when submitting grants to a major funder, we would recommend including a statistician in the planning process for your study as planning such large-scale, complex studies goes beyond the scope of this book.

16.7   Follow Up Tests

As with the one-way analysis of variance, this test produces a single overall conclusion as to whether there are any differences among the time points or study conditions. If you obtain a significant result, it is likely that you will wish to determine which condition differs from which other. This can be achieved by carrying out separate tests on whichever pairs of conditions you wish to consider. In this setting, you would use Wilcoxon signed rank tests for each of the pairs of observations that you wish to examine – for example, baseline to 1 week and baseline to three months. This would entail multiple testing (two tests in the example just given) and so, to guard against inflating the risk of false positives, you would apply the Bonferroni correction – in the example scenario, this would reduce the target P-value to 0.025 (See Section 5.2.3).

16.8   Carrying Out the Tests

See a video listed at the end of this chapter for detailed instructions on using SPSS to carry out the Friedman and follow up tests.

16.9   Describing the Effect Size

16.9.1   Median or Mean Values Among the Individual Changes

You could report the medians or means among the individual changes in scores (See Table 16.3). If you need to use the mean, it is best to quote the median, point out how insensitive the median is in this context, and explain that this is why you have made additional use of the mean.

16.9.2   Split the Scale

You could reduce the scale to two ranges (high and low scores) and report the changes in numbers in one of these categories – See Section 16.3.3.

16.10   How to Report the Test

16.10.1   Methods Section

In this section, you should set out the following:

- The ordinal or continuously varying measurement used to record the endpoint for the various different times/conditions.
- The name of the statistical analysis employed (the name mentioned in the menu structure of your statistical package).

Table 16.3 Descriptive statistics for the individual changes in dental hygiene scores when comparing the pre-training period to the one week and three month time points.

Comparison	Median	Mean	SD
Pre-training vs. One week	+1	+0.56	1.18
Pre-training vs. Three months	0	+0.09	0.78

- Any follow up test used to determine which time point or condition differs from which other and any steps taken to mitigate the effects of multiple testing.
- Any options selected other than the default settings.
- The P-value that would be considered as statistically significant.
- The name of your statistical package along with its version number and supplier.

Suitable wording might be:

> The dental hygiene scores were analysed by a Friedman test implemented as the Nonparametric "K Related Samples" method in SPSS (Version 23; IBM Corporation), considering any P-value less than 0.05 as statistically significant. Two Wilcoxon signed ranks tests were used as follow-up tests for differences between the pre-training results and those at one week and at three months respectively; these tests were carried out using the, Bonferroni corrected, critical value for P of 0.025.

16.10.2 Results Section

In this section, you should set out the following:

- The sample size.
- One of the means of presenting the data discussed in Section 16.3.
- The P-value for overall statistical significance and a statement as to whether overall statistical significance was achieved.
- The P values for each of the follow up contrasts between pairs of time points and whether they were statistically significant.
- A measure of effect size.

Suitable wording might be:

> The number of subjects studied was 43. Figure 16.4 shows the mean dental hygiene scores ($\pm$ SD) at each time point. There were statistically significant differences among the various time points (P = 0.001). Wilcoxon signed rank tests showed a statistically significant change in scores between pre-training and one week (P = 0.007), but the comparison between pre-training and three months was not significant (P = 0.432). The proportions of children achieving a grade of good or excellent were 49%, 72%, and 44% at the pre-training, one week, and three month time points, respectively.

16.10.3   Discussion Section

A key part of your discussion will be to compare the effect size seen in your work against the minimum clinically/practically relevant difference. You will need to provide and justify a value for the latter.

Nonparametric methods do not generate a confidence interval for the effect size; however, there are a number of options for discussing significance and effect size. Some suggestions follow.

- For a non-significant result: If sample sizes are small, be wary of saying there is no effect; one may be present but you have failed to detect it. With large samples, you can more safely say that there is either no effect or, at the very least, any effect is very small and therefore probably not of any practical relevance.
- For a significant result: Discuss whether the effect size is great enough to be of practical consequence and its implications for public policy or professional practice.

Rowe (2015, section 21.2.5)[1] discusses in detail the interpretation of a statistically significant finding with a nonparametric test.

16.11   Relevant Videos etc.

The following are available at
www.wiley.com/go/Mackridge/APracticalApproachtoUsingStatisticsin
HealthResearch

Video_1.1_SPSS_Basics: The absolute basics of using SPSS
Video_16.1_Friedman: Using SPSS to perform Friedman's test and
   follow up tests

SPSS data files

SPSS_16.1_Teeth: The data for the example used to illustrate this
   chapter.

Spreadsheets

Spreadsheet_16.1_Teeth: The data for the example used to illustrate
   this chapter.

---

[1] Rowe P. Essential statistics for the pharmaceutical sciences, 2nd edn. Chichester: Wiley, 2015.

17

Pearson Correlation

Pearson correlation, or simply "Correlation" as it is widely known, is used where the following circumstances apply:

- The factor is a continuously varying measurement.
- The outcome is a continuously varying measurement.
- A scatter plot of the factor and outcome shows a broadly linear relationship with no outliers or clustering.

As an example for Pearson correlation, consider a survey of lung function and how it may have been affected by the length of time for which individuals have been employed in a local cotton factory. The study involves 87 men aged 40–45 living in the area surrounding the factory. In this example, the factor and outcome are:

- Factor: The period of employment in the factory measured in years (if never, recorded as zero).
- Outcome: The participants' lung function, measured as Forced Expiratory Volume in one second (FEV1), recorded in liters.

The dataset is available from the Excel spreadsheet or SPSS data file listed at the end of this chapter.

17.1   Presenting the Data

You would almost certainly present the data in the form of a scatterplot as in Figure 17.1. Graphs like this are always described as showing

A Practical Approach to Using Statistics in Health Research: From Planning to Reporting,
First Edition. Adam Mackridge and Philip Rowe.
© 2018 John Wiley & Sons, Inc. Published 2018 by John Wiley & Sons, Inc.
Companion website: www.wiley.com/go/Mackridge/
APracticalApproachtoUsingStatisticsinHealthResearch

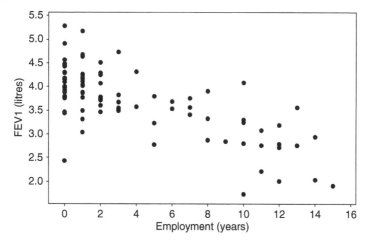

Figure 17.1 FEV1 values (liters) among residents versus number of years employment in a local cotton mill.

the outcome versus the factor. This is therefore FEV1 versus years, not vice versa.

As described in Section 4.4.2, you would use Figure 17.1 to check that the relationship is approximately linear, that there are no outliers, and that the data do not form distinct clusters. In this example, the figure does not indicate any problems, and Pearson correlation is appropriate.

17.2 Correlation Coefficient and Statistical Significance

The closeness of the relationship between the factor and outcome is expressed as the correlation coefficient (r). This can take any value between −1 and +1, with the extreme values representing perfect negative correlation (−1; one value falls, while the other rises) or perfect positive correlation (+1; the factor & outcome both rise together) and zero meaning no relationship whatsoever. If you added a trend line to a graph such as Figure 17.1, cases with strong correlation (r value close to −1 or +1) would have all the points adhering very closely to the trend line. With an r value close to zero, the points would be scattered on both sides of the line.

The significance test is heavily influenced by the strength of correlation (stronger correlation giving greater likelihood of significance), but it will also take account of the sample size. It is therefore possible that even weak correlation (r close to zero) may be deemed statistically significant if there is a very large amount of data. For a fuller description of the interpretation of r and testing its significance, see our sister publication (Rowe 2015).[1]

In our example, r = −0.723, and the relationship is statistically significant, with P<0.001.

The video listed at the end of this chapter shows how to use SPSS to perform Pearson correlation analysis.

17.3   Planning Sample Sizes

To plan your sample size, you will need the following:

- The smallest degree of correlation you want to be able to detect – this is expressed as a value for the correlation coefficient.
- The power you wish to achieve – typically, 90% is satisfactory for most health-related studies.
- The P-value you will consider as statistically significant. Most statistical packages use a default value of 0.05. The program may refer to this as "Alpha" – see glossary.

Necessary sample sizes can then be determined using G*Power. For example, if you want 90% power to detect a correlation coefficient of either +0.5 or −0.5 (or stronger), you will need a sample size of 37. A video listed at the end of this chapter shows how to use G*Power to calculate sample sizes for correlation.

17.4   Effect Size and Practical Relevance

A bare report that the correlation coefficient is −0.723, as with our example, is not particularly informative as it only gives the reader information about the closeness of the relationship between the factor and outcome and gives no indication of the relevance of this relationship in real life.

---

[1] Rowe P. Essential statistics for the pharmaceutical sciences, 2nd edn. Chichester: Wiley, 2015.

Including a figure, such as Figure 17.1, accompanied by an interpretation of the clinical or practical relevance of the relationship, will help the reader to appreciate the importance (or otherwise) of the finding.

For a correlation relationship to have practical relevance, you need to establish that both of the following are true:

- The outcome value varies over a range that is wide enough to be practically, or clinically relevant
- The factor being investigated accounts for a considerable proportion of the variation in the outcome

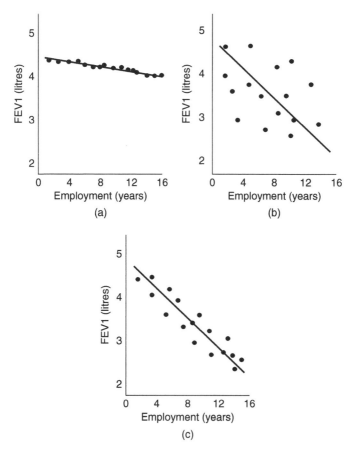

Figure 17.2 Possible relationships between FEV1 and period of employment in a cotton factory.

Figure 17.2 shows relationships using three sets of data exploring the years of employment versus FEV1 question.

In Figure 17.2a, the r value would be close to −1, showing very strong correlation, but there is so little difference in FEV1 between those with short and long periods of employment, that it is not likely to be of any great practical relevance – i.e. working in this factory for a long period will result in a very small decline in lung function – so small that it is not be likely to be of real concern.

In part b, there is plenty of variation in FEV1, but the correlation is low (plotted values are scattered across the graph, rather than being close to the trend line), and even those individuals with long periods of employment may have values considerably greater than those with only brief employment. In this scenario, some individuals show sufficient decline in lung function to be of concern, but the time worked in the factory is not well correlated to this, suggesting that some other factor is at play. In such a scenario, it would be appropriate to investigate this further to work out what really is impacting on the participants' health.

In part c, there is both a clinically relevant decline in lung function over time AND there is a strong correlation between the factor and outcome, indicating that the time worked in the factory has a strong association with this marked decline in lung function. In this case, it would be appropriate to take steps to mitigate the risks for workers in the factory to minimize any impact on health.

17.5 Regression

It is possible to go a step beyond correlation and perform a regression analysis. This does everything that correlation does, but also produces an equation that could be used to predict FEV1 from the numbers of years of employment. In our worked example, the regression formula is:

$$FEV1 = 4.16 - 0.116 \times Years$$

This equation can be useful in quantifying the extent to which the factor under investigation influences your outcome, and this may then be helpful in designing practical interventions. In the current example, on average, one year's additional employment in the factory will be associated with a decline in FEV1 of 0.116 liters, and this could help to inform discussions concerning the need for changed factory regulations, or in the case of a retrospective analysis, a claim for compensation!

The video listed at the end of this chapter shows how to add a regression analysis.

17.6 How to Report the Analysis

17.6.1 Methods

You should include all of the following:

- How your sample size was calculated. (If it was not pre-calculated, say why not; maybe all available cases in a pre-existing database were used.)
- The two measured variables (factor and outcome).
- The name of the statistical analysis employed (use the exact same wording as that in the menu structure of the package you used).
- Options selected (if any are different form the program's defaults).
- The P-value that would be considered as statistically significant.
- If additional regression analysis was used, it needs to be mentioned.
- The name of your statistical package along with its version number and supplier.

Suitable wording might be:

A minimum sample size of 37 was determined using G*Power (version 3.1; Heinrich-Heine-Universität, Düsseldorf). This was designed to detect a correlation coefficient of ±0.5 or stronger *(give references or justification)*, with a power of 90% and an a priori P-value of <0.05. Correlation and regression analyses of FEV1 values and years of employment were carried out using SPSS (Version 23; IBM Corporation).

17.6.2 Results

You should include all of the following:

- The sample size used in the analysis.
- A clearly labeled scatterplot.
- The correlation coefficient (r).

- The P-value and a statement as to whether statistical significance was achieved.
- The regression equation, if this analysis was added.

Suitable wording might be:

> A total of 87 cases were included in the analysis, and these demonstrated a statistically significant ($p < 0.001$) negative correlation ($r = -0.713$) between FEV1 and years of work (Figure 17.1). The regression equation was: FEV1 = 4.16 − 0.116 x Years, indicating that each additional year of working in the factory was associated with a reduction in FEV1 of 0.116 litres.

17.6.3 Discussion

A key part of your discussion will concern the practical relevance of any correlation detected (See Sections 6.5 and 6.6).

- For a non-significant result: If sample sizes are small, be wary of saying there is no effect; one may be present but you have failed to detect it. With large samples, you can more safely say that there is either no effect or, at the very least, any effect is very small and therefore probably not of any practical relevance.
- For a significant result: Discuss whether the effect size is great enough to be of practical consequence and its implications for public policy or professional practice.

17.7 Relevant Videos etc.

The following are available at
www.wiley.com/go/Mackridge/APracticalApproachtoUsingStatisticsin
Health Research

Videos

Video_1.1_SPSS_Basics: The absolute basics of using SPSS
Video_17.1_PearsonCorrelationRegression: Using SPSS to carry out Pearson correlation and regression analyses
Video_17.2_Pearson_SampSize: Calculating the sample size required for Pearson Correlation using G*Power

SPSS data files

SPSS_17.1_FEV1VersusYears: The data for the example used to illustrate this chapter.

Spreadsheets

Spreadsheet_17.1_FEV1VersusYears.xlsx: The data for the example used to illustrate this chapter.

18

Spearman Correlation

The appropriate circumstances for using Spearman correlation are discussed in detail in Chapter 4. The example to be discussed in this chapter concerns the effect of age on satisfaction among new mothers concerning a maternity service. The factor and outcome are thus:

- Factor: A continuously varying measurement – Age measured in years.
- Outcome: Ordinal data – Assessments of satisfaction using a scale (1 = Strongly dissatisfied; 2 = Dissatisfied; 3 = Neutral; 4 = Generally Satisfied; 5=Very satisfied).

In this case, Spearman correlation is preferred to Pearson's, because one of the measures (the outcome) is ordinal. The data set is available from a spreadsheet or SPSS data file listed at the end of this chapter

A video listed at the end of this chapter shows how to use SPSS to perform Spearman correlation analysis.

18.1 Presenting the Data

A scatterplot is unlikely to work satisfactorily, as the satisfaction scores can take only five values, hence it is likely that several dots will coincide and only one point will show. In Figure 18.1, participants have been divided into four approximately equally sized groups based on age, and within each group, we have the proportions who provided the various satisfaction gradings. The figure only shows the proportions in

A Practical Approach to Using Statistics in Health Research: From Planning to Reporting,
First Edition. Adam Mackridge and Philip Rowe.
© 2018 John Wiley & Sons, Inc. Published 2018 by John Wiley & Sons, Inc.
Companion website: www.wiley.com/go/Mackridge/
APracticalApproachtoUsingStatisticsinHealthResearch

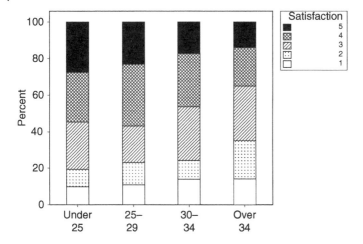

Figure 18.1 Proportions of new mothers in four age bands who provided varioussatisfaction ratings for the maternity service (1 = Strongly dissatisfied; 2 = Dissatisfied; 3 = Neutral; 4 = Generally satisfied; 5 = Very satisfied).

each category, not the absolute numbers, thus the figure would need to be accompanied by a report of the sample sizes for each age range.

18.2   Testing for Evidence of Inappropriate Distributions

As described in Chapter 4, correlation is not applicable to some data relationships, so it is important to check that the current data is appropriate. If your data produces scatter plots that resemble any of those shown in Figure 18.2, then it is likely that no correlation method will be appropriate. Figure 18.2a shows a non-monotonic relationship while part b shows distinct clusters.

18.3   Rho and Statistical Significance

Spearman correlation produces a correlation coefficient (rho) that ranges from −1 to +1, with the extreme values representing perfect relatedness between the factor and outcome and zero showing no relationship at all. The rho correlation coefficient from the current example is −0.156 with

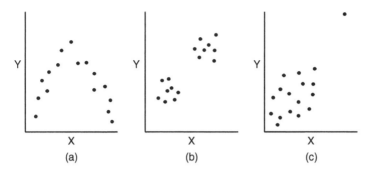

Figure 18.2 Data relationships that would not be suitable for Spearman correlation.

a P-value of 0.015, so there is statistically significant evidence of a negative relationship (less favorable opinions among mothers of greater age).

18.4   An Outline of the Significance Test

Two aspects of the data will determine whether your results are statistically significant:

- The strength of correlation. (Remember that rho values close to either +1 or −1 constitute strong correlation; it is rho values near zero that are likely to prove non-significant.)
- The size of your samples: Large samples are more likely to be significant than small ones.

18.5   Planning Sample Sizes

To plan your sample size, you will need the following:

- The smallest degree of correlation you want to be able to detect – this is expressed as a value for the correlation coefficient.
- The power you wish to achieve – typically, 90% is satisfactory for most health-related studies.
- The P-value you will consider as statistically significant. Most statistical packages use a default value of 0.05. The program may refer to this as "Alpha" – see glossary.

Necessary sample sizes for a Pearson correlation can then be determined using G*Power. However, the Spearman method may be somewhat less powerful than Pearson's so the indicated sample size should be increased by about 20%. For example, if you want 90% power to detect a correlation coefficient of either +0.25 or −0.25 (or stronger) using Pearson correlation, G*Power will indicate a sample size of 164. This should be increased to around 200 for the Spearman method. A video listed at the end of this chapter shows how to use G*Power to calculate sample sizes for correlation.

18.6   Effect Size

There are a few ways that you might use to describe the effect size. Which one is most appropriate will depend on the particular circumstances of your study.

The rho value of −0.156 provides a measure of effect size. The value is quite close to zero, so the relationship cannot be very strong, but it is difficult to use this value to assess quite how strongly age affects women's opinions. In Figure 18.1, the participants have been divided into four approximately equally sized groups based on age. The proportions providing each response are then shown for each group. This allows the reader to see the extent of the change in ratings across the four age ranges.

You could consider describing the four age groups in terms of their median or mean values. As is generally the case, medians of five-point ordinal scales are not very informative; the medians for the four groups are 4, 4, 3, and 3 as we pass from the youngest to the oldest groups, but this does little to clarify the strength of the relationship. You could quote the means for each age group, quoting the lack of sensitivity of the medians as your reason for using the means.

Finally, you might consider that a grade of at least "Generally satisfied" should be a target and report the proportions giving one of the two top grades – for our example, these are 55, 57, 47, and 35% as we go from the youngest to the oldest group.

18.7   Where Both Measures Are Ordinal

18.7.1   Educational Level and Willingness to Undertake Internet Research – An Example Where Both Measures Are Ordinal

Spearman correlation can also be applied in cases where you want to look for a relationship between two measures that are both ordinal.

For example, we might want to relate educational level and likelihood of seeking information on psoriasis using the Internet. These would be measured as levels of education (1 = Nothing beyond age 16; 2 = Up to age 18; 3 = Undergraduate degree or equivalent; 4 = Postgraduate qualification) and likelihood of Internet use (1 = Definitely no; 2 = Unlikely; 3 = Likely; 4 = Definitely yes).

The data set is available as an Excel spreadsheet or as an SPSS data file listed at the end of this chapter.

18.7.2   Presenting the Data

Section 18.1 pointed out that it is generally very difficult to represent data as a scatterplot when one parameter is continuous measured and the other ordinal. When both parameters are ordinal, it is hopeless. Typically, the results are presented as either a table or a graph (See Table 18.1 and Figure 18.3), but as can be seen from these examples, a graphical representation often helps the reader to observe any patterns in the data more easily.

Figure 18.3 only describes the proportions in each category, not the absolute numbers; thus, the figure would need to be accompanied by a report of the sample sizes for each educational level.

18.7.3   Rho and Statistical Significance

The rho correlation coefficient from the current example is +0.276 with a P-value of < 0.001, so there is statistically significant evidence that likelihood of internet searching is influenced positively by level of education.

Table 18.1 Numbers and proportions with various levels of likelihood of using the internet to research psoriasis among groups separated by level of education (1 Lowest; 4 Highest).

	Educational level 1	Educational level 2	Educational level 3	Educational level 4
Definitely No	10 (11%)	11 (11%)	5 (5%)	1 (2%)
Unlikely	37 (42%)	15 (15%)	21 (22%)	9 (14%)
Likely	27 (30%)	42 (40%)	36 (38%)	21 (33%)
Definitely Yes	15 (17%)	35 (34%)	34 (35%)	32 (51%)

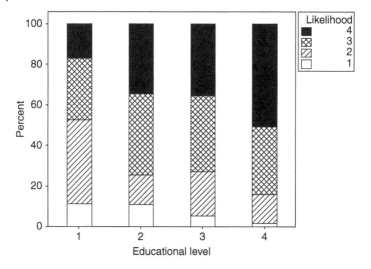

Figure 18.3 Proportions with various levels of willingness to research psoriasis on the Internet among four groups separated according to educational level (1 Lowest; 4 Highest).

18.7.4   Effect Size

The rho value of +0.276 is a measure of effect size. The value is reasonably strong, so the relationship is quite marked, but it is difficult to use this value to assess quite how strongly education affects use of the Internet. Figure 18.3 allows the reader to see the extent of the change in likelihoods across four educational ranges.

18.8   How to Report Spearman Correlation Analyses

What follows would be suitable for reporting either of the examples considered in this chapter.

18.8.1   Methods

You should include all of the following:

- How your sample size was calculated. (If it was not pre-calculated, say why not; maybe all available cases in a pre-existing database were used.)

- The two measures (continuous measured or ordinal) that were considered.
- The name of the statistical analysis employed (use the exact same wording as that in the menu structure of the package you used).
- Options selected (if any are different form the program's defaults).
- The P-value that would be considered as statistically significant.
- The name of your statistical package along with its version number and supplier.

In the case of the study into women's ages and satisfaction scores, suitable wording might be:

> A minimum sample size of 200 was determined using the method described in Mackridge and Rowe (2018). This was based on a target of a Spearman correlation coefficient (rho) of ±0.25 or greater being detectable *(give references or justification)*, a power of 90%, and an a priori P value of <0.05. A correlation analysis between satisfaction and age was carried out using SPSS, selecting Spearman correlation (Version 23; IBM Corporation).

18.8.2 Results

You should include all of the following:

- Sample size used
- A figure similar to Figure 18.1 or 18.3.
- If both measures are ordinal, you could use a table such as Table 18.1 in place of Figure 18.3.
- The Spearman correlation coefficient (rho).
- The P-value and a statement as to whether statistical significance was achieved.

Suitable wording for the age/satisfaction study might be:

> A total of 244 cases were included in the analysis. There was a statistically significant (p = 0.015), but weak, negative relationship (rho = −0.156) between women's age and their satisfaction with maternity services. Figure 18.1 shows participants divided into four approximately equally sized groups based on age and indicates the proportions expressing varying levels of satisfaction in each group.

18.8.3 Discussion

A key part of your discussion will concern the practical relevance of any correlation detected, referring to the effect size using any of the methods described in Section 18.6.

- For a non-significant result: If sample sizes are small, be wary of saying there is no effect; one may be present but you have failed to detect it. With large samples, you can more safely say that there is either no effect or, at the very least, any effect is very small and therefore probably not of any practical relevance.
- For a significant result: Discuss whether the effect size is great enough to be of practical consequence and its implications for public policy or professional practice.

18.9 Relevant Videos etc.

The following are available at www.wiley.com/go/Mackridge/APracticalApproachtoUsingStatisticsin HealthResearch

Videos

Video_1.1_SPSS_Basics: The absolute basics of using SPSS
Video_17.2_Pearson_SampSize: Calculating the sample size required for Pearson Correlation using G*Power
Video_18.1_SpearmanCorrelation: Using SPSS to carry out Spearman correlation

SPSS data files

SPSS_18.1_SatisVersusAge: The data for the first example used to illustrate this chapter.
SPSS_18.2_InternetVersusEducation: The data for the second example used to illustrate this chapter.

Spreadsheets

Spreadsheet_18.1_SatisVersusAge: The data for the first example used to illustrate this chapter.
Spreadsheet_18.2_InternetVersusEducation: The data for the second example used to illustrate this chapter.

19

Logistic Regression

19.1   Use of Logistic Regression with Categorical Outcomes

In this book, we will only discuss logistic regression for categorical outcomes that have two possible values, hence the term "Binary logistic regression." Other forms of logistic regression go beyond the scope of the simple-to-use statistics that this book focuses upon. See our sister text (Rowe 2015)[1] for details of other forms of logistic regression.

Binary logistic regression is used where the following circumstances apply:

• The factor is an ordinal or continuously varying measurement.
• The outcome is categorical, with **two** possible values.

The worked example we will use concerns the relationship between daily dose of drug and whether or not patients experience a particular side-effect – in this case, gallstones. The purpose of this study is to evaluate if there is a dose-response relationship for an apparent adverse drug reaction. We have pooled several sets of medical records to identify a large group (over 1500) of patients who have been using the drug for more than two years and have data on the daily dose taken, their body weights, and whether there has been a new diagnosis

---
[1]   Rowe P. Essential statistics for the pharmaceutical sciences, 2nd edn. Chichester: Wiley, 2015.

A Practical Approach to Using Statistics in Health Research: From Planning to Reporting, First Edition. Adam Mackridge and Philip Rowe.
© 2018 John Wiley & Sons, Inc. Published 2018 by John Wiley & Sons, Inc.
Companion website: www.wiley.com/go/Mackridge/
APracticalApproachtoUsingStatisticsinHealthResearch

of gallstones within the last two years. The factor and outcome are thus:

- Factor: Daily dose of drug (mg per kg body weight per day).
- Outcome: diagnosis of gallstones (Yes/No).

The dataset is available as a spreadsheet and an SPSS data file and a video shows how to perform binary logistic regression using SPSS. These are all listed at the end of this chapter.

19.2   An Outline of the Significance Test

Figure 19.1 shows two possible relationships between a binary outcome and a measured factor, using the current example of drug dose affecting the risk of gallstones.

Two aspects of the data will determine whether your results are statistically significant:

- The nature of the relationship:
  – Figure 19.1a shows an example of a strong relationship. The proportion of positive cases suddenly increases from virtually zero to almost one hundred percent at a critical value of the continuous measured factor (Drug dose). This critical value can therefore demarcate most of the positive from the negative cases. A set of results like this is very likely to be statistically significant. In addition, this type of relationship is likely to be clinically or practically relevant.
  – Figure 19.1b shows a much weaker relationship. There is only a gradual increase in the proportion of positive cases as the factor (Dose) increases, and the proportion only changes over a relatively narrow range. There is certainly no critical value for the dose that sharply demarcates between positive and negative cases. This data is much less likely to be statistically significant; it is also less likely that the findings will have clinical or practical relevance.
- The size of your samples: Large samples are more likely to return a significant result than small ones.

19.3   Planning Sample Sizes

Attempting an exact determination of necessary sample size for logistic regression for the sort of project envisaged by this book is

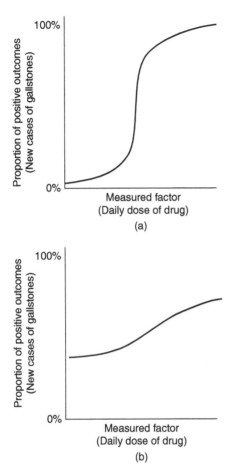

Figure 19.1 (a) A strong relationship between a binary outcome and a continuously varying measured factor, which is likely to be statistically significant. (b) A weaker relationship that is less likely to be significant.

unrealistic. The amount of data you will need depends upon how strong a relationship you can realistically expect to see between the measured factor and the categorical outcome that you intend to investigate. With a strong relationship such as that shown in Figure 19.1a, a relatively small sample size (say 50) would suffice. However, with a weak relationship such as part b of the same figure, a sample of 1000 might be needed. Therefore, you should use any information available to estimate the expected strength of the relationship and tailor your sample size within the above range.

19.4   Results of the Analysis

The question being asked is whether there is convincing evidence that the probability that a patient will develop gallstones is related to drug dosage. The logistic regression yields a P-value of 0.016, so there is statistically significant evidence of a relationship. Your computer output will also include a value for the odds ratio (68.2). Any value for the odds ratio that is greater than 1.0 tells you that higher values for the factor (larger doses) are associated with greater likelihoods of the event (gallstones). Values of less than 1.0 imply the opposite pattern (greater doses associated with less likelihood of gallstones). Interpreting the actual value of the odds ratio can be problematic – see the discussion in the next section.

19.5   Describing the Effect Size

The traditional measure of effect size for logistic regression is the odds ratio. The concept of an odds ratio was explained in Section 7.9.4, but in short, it is essentially the change in the likelihood of the event if you increase the factor by one unit. In our example, the odds ratio is 68.2, which means that if two patients had dose sizes that differed by one unit (1 mg/kg/day), the patient with the higher dose would be at 68 times greater risk of gallstones compared to the patient with the lower dose. However, this is misleading as the actual values for daily dose only vary over the range of 0.193 to 0.65 mg/kg/day, so in fact the largest difference observed is actually 0.459 mg/kg/day. The notion of two patients with doses that differed by 1 mg/kg/day is quite unrealistic.

   You should normally report the odds ratio, but you can also present the data in some other format to help the reader understand it more clearly. One approach is to divide the cases into ranges based on the values of the measured factor (Dose in this case) and report the event rate in each group. In Figure 19.2, the cases have been separated into four groups with equal numbers in each group. The first group contains all the cases with a dose size smaller than the first quartile, the

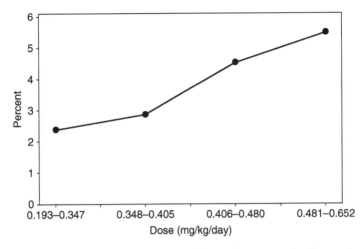

Figure 19.2 Percentage of patients developing a new case of gallstones during the two years of the study. Patients have been divided into four groups based on dosage of drug received.

next contains all those with a dose between the first and second quartile, and so on.

The figure successfully conveys the information that there is a dose-response relationship, and it also shows the effect size: patients taking the highest dose run just over twice the risk of gallstones compared to those on the lowest doses. The advantage of this approach is that it describes the increased risk over the actual range of doses used, whereas the odds ratio was trying to describe the effect of an unrealistically large dose change (1 mg/day/kg).

19.6 How to Report the Analysis

19.6.1 Methods

You should include all of the following:

- The continuous measured variable that was considered as a possible factor.
- The binary categorical variable that formed the outcome.
- Which of the two potential outcomes was considered as the "Event."

- The name of the statistical analysis employed (use the exact same wording as that in the menu structure of the package you used).
- Options selected (if any are different form the program's defaults).
- The P-value that would be considered as statistically significant.
- The name of your statistical package along with its version number and supplier.

Suitable wording might be:

> Binary logistic regression was performed, taking dose (in mg/kg/day) as the factor and the presence or absence of a new case of gallstones as the binary outcome, with positive cases of gallstones being treated as the event. The analysis was performed using SPSS (Version 23; IBM Corporation), with an a priori value of P<0.05 being taken to indicate statistical significance.

19.6.2   Results

You should include all of the following:

- Sample size used.
- The P-value and a statement as to whether statistical significance was achieved.
- The odds ratio.
- A figure similar to 19.2.

Suitable wording might be:

> A total of 1680 cases were used in the analysis, which showed a statistically significant relationship between dose and the likelihood of a new case of gallstones (P = 0.016). The odds ratio was 68.2 for a 1 mg/kg/day increase in dose. Figure 19.2 shows the patients divided into four equally sized groups based on dose size, and indicates the likelihood of disease in each group. It demonstrates that the risk is around twice as high with the greatest doses compared to the lowest.

19.6.3   Discussion

Your discussion may need to clarify how to interpret the odds ratio (OR). In the current case, you would need to emphasize that the OR takes such a high value because it is considering an unrealistically large change in dose.

A key part of your discussion will be to compare any effect size seen in your work against the minimum clinically/practically relevant difference. You will need to provide and justify a value for the latter.

- For a non-significant result: If sample sizes are small, be wary of saying there is no effect; one may be present but you have failed to detect it. With large samples, you can more safely say that there is either no effect or, at the very least, any effect is very small and therefore probably not of any practical relevance.
- For a significant result: Discuss whether the effect size is great enough to be of practical consequence and its implications for public policy or professional practice.

19.7   Relevant Videos etc.

The following are available at
www.wiley.com/go/Mackridge/APracticalApproachtoUsingStatisticsin
HealthResearch

Videos

Video_1.1_SPSS_Basics: The absolute basics of using SPSS
Video_19.1_LogisticRegression: Using SPSS for binary logistic regression

SPSS data files

SPSS_19.1_DoseVersusGallStones: The data for the example used to illustrate this chapter.

Spreadsheets

Spreadsheet_19.1_DoseVersusGallStones: The data for the example used to illustrate this chapter.

20

Cronbach's Alpha

20.1   Appropriate Situations for the Use of Cronbach's Alpha

If you have a series of questions each producing a score on an ordinal scale, you might want to combine them all to produce a single overall score. The validity of combining the results may rest upon an assumption that all the questions are essentially measuring the same thing, and that assumption would need to be tested. If the questions do indeed all measure the same thing, then the responses should be correlated. An example of such a correlation can be seen in the AUDIT tool for assessing risk associated with alcohol consumption. The questions in this tool concern number of drinking sessions per week, how much is drunk per session, problems with remembering events while drinking, etc. If an individual is drinking in a risky manner, then nearly all the questions will generate high scores, but someone whose alcohol consumption behavior has lower risk will generate a series of low scores. We would therefore expect to see a high level of correlation – individuals producing a high score to one question would be expected to generate many other high scores, and similarly a person with a low score to one question will generate generally low scores.

The usual measure of this form of correlation is Cronbach's Alpha. Like most correlation measures, this could theoretically take any value between −1 and +1. However, negative values are unlikely as these would only arise if those who produced a high score for one question systematically produced low scores for others and vice versa, and

A Practical Approach to Using Statistics in Health Research: From Planning to Reporting, First Edition. Adam Mackridge and Philip Rowe.
© 2018 John Wiley & Sons, Inc. Published 2018 by John Wiley & Sons, Inc.
Companion website: www.wiley.com/go/Mackridge/
APracticalApproachtoUsingStatisticsinHealthResearch

the author of the questions is unlikely to be so far off the mark as to produce negative correlations. Therefore, the usual range is zero (no relationship whatsoever) to +1, the maximum value arising only if each individual gives completely consistent responses, i.e. their score for every question was one, or all questions were scored as two, etc.

One situation where responses should be very highly correlated (values very close to +1) is where a series of questions are essentially asking the same thing, but are worded differently. This might be done in the hope that the mean score from two or three essentially identical questions will reflect the true situation more reliably than a single question; the effect of any occasional aberrant responses should be diluted out by other more carefully considered responses. It would also be appropriate to calculate Cronbach's Alpha in this situation.

20.2   Inappropriate Uses of Alpha

There are situations where it makes perfect sense to combine the responses to several questions into a single score, but there would be no expectation of correlation among the responses. An example would be the production of a score for overall satisfaction with a service. Questions might be asked about waiting times, clarity of instructions, staff friendliness, accessibility for people with disabilities, and so on – all validly contributing to patient satisfaction, but with no reason why positive responses to one question would be accompanied by positive answers to any other.

> Use Cronbach's Alpha selectively. Use it only when the rationale for combining several scores depends upon the responses being correlated.

20.3   Interpretation

It is commonly said that Alpha needs to take a minimum value of 0.7. That figure provides a reasonable guide, but is somewhat arbitrary. The figure that might reasonably be attained will depend on context. If you are simply asking the same question in reworded formats (as in the last paragraph of Section 20.1), 0.7 would be a pretty unambitious target.

If Alpha takes a very high value, the response to any one of the questions will quite reliably predict the responses to all the others. Under these circumstances, there would be little purpose in asking numerous questions. If the high Alpha value was based on just two or three questions, there is no great issue, but if it was based on a long series of questions, you could remove some with almost no loss of information (and make life easier for your respondents).

20.4 Reverse Scoring

Typically, each question may present a statement that brings Likert responses that are scored as: Strongly disagree = 1; Disagree = 2; Neutral = 3; Agree = 4; Strongly agree = 5. However, in a well-designed survey, some statements are worded positively and others negatively to reduce the risk of acquiescence bias, and this can present a complication if scored using the above format. For instance, we might have the statements:

- I nearly always remembered to take the tablets (**high** scores = better adherence).
- It was easy to take the tablets regularly (**high** scores = better adherence).
- There were quite a few days where I forgot to take the tablets (**low** scores = better adherence).

The respondent should consistently report either good or poor adherence. However, if all the responses are converted to numerical values as suggested above, the results from the third question will be negatively correlated with the others. The appropriate action is to reverse the scores for the final question: Strongly disagree would be coded as 5 and Strongly agree as 1. Higher scores then always indicate better adherence, and all three sets of responses should be positively correlated.

20.5 An Example

The example is 34 patients' responses to the three statements in Section 20.4, with the addition of a fourth statement:
- I have good medicines adherence.

The results are available from the MS Excel spreadsheet or SPSS data file listed at the end of the chapter. The responses to the third statement are recorded as "Q3Rev" because the response scores have been reversed as described in Section 20.4.

20.6   Performing and Interpreting the Analysis

Typically, your results will be stored with the responses to each question in their own data column (four in the current case). When analyzing this in a software package, it is possible (and advisable) to add a series of additional analyses where each question is removed one at a time.

The video listed at the end of the chapter shows how to execute the analysis.

The example data set produces an Alpha value of 0.605. Under most circumstances, this would be considered (at best) a rather marginal result. In this specific context (four statements all saying the same thing), it is disappointing.

The results of omitting each question in turn are shown in Table 20.1.

The table shows that if Alpha is calculated without question 1 (retaining the final three), Alpha is 0.253 and then if we use all except question 2, it is 0.402, and so on. The striking feature is that when question four is omitted, Alpha suddenly increases to a very respectable 0.893. The interpretation would be that the first three questions are well correlated, but number four is poorly correlated with the

Table 20.1 Cronbach's Alpha values when each question was omitted one at a time.

Question omitted	Alpha
Q1	0.253
Q2	0.402
Q3Rev	0.339
Q4	0.893

other three. That should trigger a particularly close re-assessment of that question. On relooking at the fourth question, it becomes clear that the statement was badly worded: the use of a technical term "medicines adherence" will be unfamiliar to many patients and has led to inconsistency in their responses.

20.7 How to Report Cronbach's Alpha Analyses

Typically, in smaller studies, Cronbach's Alpha analysis is used in developing a series of questions for a survey, and preliminary data will be obtained by piloting these questions. In such circumstances, you would report all aspects of this in your methods section using wording along the lines of "The questionnaire was piloted with 50 individuals not included in the sample for the current study, and the scale was determined to have a Cronbach's Alpha of 0.78, following removal of two statements."

However, if you are designing and validating a new survey or clinical evaluation tool that you hope will be used by others to measure some behavioral, attitudinal, or clinical feature of respondents, you would describe the various aspects in the usual sections described below.

20.7.1 Methods Section

You should include all of the following:

- How statements were scored (e.g. Strongly disagree = 1; Disagree = 2; Neutral = 3; Agree = 4; Strongly agree = 5).
- How negatively worded phrases were scored and which statements were negative.
- The name of the statistical analysis employed (use the exact same wording as that in the menu structure of the package you used).
- Options selected (if any are different from the program's defaults).
- The value of Alpha that would be considered as acceptable for correlation to be confirmed.
- The name of your statistical package along with its version number and supplier.

In the case of the study into medicines adherence described above, suitable wording might be:

> Responses to questions with positive statements (indicating better adherence) were scored as: Strongly disagree = 1; Disagree = 2; Neutral = 3; Agree = 4; Strongly agree = 5. Those with negatively phrased statements, indicating poorer adherence, (Q3) were reverse scored (Strongly agree = 1 to Strongly disagree = 5). A reliability analysis of responses to all four questions was carried out using SPSS, selecting Cronbach's Alpha (Version 23; IBM Corporation). Calculation of alpha values with sequential deletion of items was added. A Cronbach's Alpha value of >0.7 was taken as indicating acceptable correlation.

20.7.2   Results

You should include all of the following:

- A table similar to Table 20.1.
- A description of any statements that needed to be excluded from the calculation of the final aggregate score.
- The Cronbach's Alpha value for the final aggregate score.
- The nature of any aggregate scores that were calculated from the data (including minimum and maximum scores and their meanings).

Suitable wording for the medicines adherence study might be:

> Responses from a total of 34 participants were included in the analysis. Calculation of Cronbach's Alpha revealed that the statement in question four poorly correlated with statements in the other questions, and this was excluded. The Adherence Score, calculated as the sum of the responses to questions one to three, produced a correlation of 0.893 (Cronbach's Alpha). The Adherence Scores ranged from 3 (indicating poor adherence) through to 15 (indicating excellent adherence).

20.7.3   Discussion

A key part of your discussion will be to explain why excluded statements were poorly correlated; typically, where validating a new tool/survey, additional data would have been collected to understand the respondents' interpretation of the statements to help with this. In cases where such poor correlation cannot be explained, it may be taken to indicate a problem in the design of the tool or the validation mechanism(s) employed and would lay the whole series of statements, or the concept of measuring whatever feature is of interest, open to question.

20.7   Relevant Videos etc.

The following are available at
www.wiley.com/go/Mackridge/APracticalApproachtoUsingStatisticsin
HealthResearch

Videos

Video_1.1_SPSS_Basics: The absolute basics of using SPSS
Video_20.1_Cronbach: Using SPSS to calculate Cronbach's Alpha, including sequential removal of each item

SPSS data files

SPSS_20.1_Cronbach: The data for the example used to illustrate this chapter.

Spreadsheets

Spreadsheet_20.1_Cronbach.xlsx: The data for the example used to illustrate this chapter.

Glossary

Word	Meaning
Absolute risk difference (ARD)	The risk (likelihood of a particular outcome) in the experimental or exposed group minus that in the control or unexposed group.
Acquiescence bias	A form of response bias that is seen in surveys and other research with human participants whereby they indicate a stronger agreement with something than reality – essentially, they don't want to be disagreeable.
Alpha	The risk that your sample(s) will lead to a false conclusion that there is statistically significant evidence of an effect when one does not exist (false positive). This is usually expressed as a P-value, with a typical cut-off being P < 0.05 equating to a 5% risk of a false positive being acceptable.
Analysis of Variance (ANOVA)	One of a family of statistical tests used when individuals are studied under different conditions or at different times and the outcome is a continuously varying measure. These tests are used where the experimental structure is more complex that that relevant for a t-test.
Bar chart	A graphical representation of the frequency and/or proportion of individuals/organizations that fall into each category when describing categorical or ordinal data. Spaces are left between bars to indicate distinct categories.
Beta	The risk that your sample(s) will fail to achieve statistical significance where a difference or effect is present (false negative). Generally due to inadequate sample sizes.

A Practical Approach to Using Statistics in Health Research: From Planning to Reporting, First Edition. Adam Mackridge and Philip Rowe.
© 2018 John Wiley & Sons, Inc. Published 2018 by John Wiley & Sons, Inc.
Companion website: www.wiley.com/go/Mackridge/
APracticalApproachtoUsingStatisticsinHealthResearch

Word	Meaning
Bimodal	Measured data that falls into two distinct clusters. There are high frequencies for both relatively high and low values, but few or no individuals with intermediate values. On a graph with a bimodal distribution you can see two "humps," rather than the usual one hump seen in a standard normal distribution.
Binary	Categorical data where there are only two, mutually exclusive outcomes, e.g. Success/Failure or Live/Dead. Same as "Dichotomous."
Bonferroni correction	A method to raise the standard of proof in each of a series of statistical tests so that each test has less than a 5% risk of producing a false positive, and the group of tests then has a joint 5% risk of a false positive.
Case : Control study	One study group contains individuals who have developed a condition and the other contains individuals who have not developed it. The study then determines what proportion of individuals in each group have a particular characteristic or had been exposed to a suspected risk factor, to attempt to retrospectively identify risk factors that may cause the condition under investigation.
Categorical data	Describes the number of people or objects that fall into each of several distinct classes. The various classes cannot be arranged into any logical order. Examples of this type of data include sex, colors, ward number, and ethnicity.
Chi-square test	Statistical test for the effect of a categorical factor upon a categorical outcome. Full name is "Contingency chi-square test."
Clinically Relevant Difference (CRD)	The smallest difference in the characteristic under study between two groups that would have any real impact on the patient. For example, a difference of 5 mmHg in blood pressure between an intervention and control group would be likely to result in clinically meaningful different outcomes for the patients in the two groups; as such, we can define this a clinically relevant difference.
Collapsing a contingency table	Combining the data from two (or more) rows or columns to simplify a contingency table. See also *Reducing a contingency table*.
Concordant	Term used in relation to McNemar's test. The data for a participant/organization is concordant if they have the same outcome under both conditions being studied.
Confidence interval (CI)	Two values that indicate the upper and lower limits of the likely true population value. These are usually quoted as 95% Confidence Intervals, where there is a 95% certainty that the true value lies in the range.

Word	Meaning
Confounding	An association between two characteristics that may falsely suggest a cause and effect relationship. For example, an association between age and likelihood of experiencing adverse drug events, where the reality is that age is associated with increasing use of medicines and this, in turn, is associated with increased risk of experiencing an adverse drug event.
Contingency chi-square test	Statistical test for the effect of a categorical factor upon a categorical outcome.
Contingency table	A table where both the columns and rows record categorized data.
Continuous measured data	Measurements that could (at least in principle) produce fractional values with any number of significant digits.
Correlation coefficient (r)	A measure of association between two sets of continuous measured data. Produced by Pearson correlation. Takes a value between −1 and +1. A plot of one value versus the other will show all points exactly on a straight line if r equals +1 or −1. With r = 0, the points are randomly scattered.
Correlation coefficient (rho)	A measure of association between two sets of measured data. Produced by Spearman correlation. Takes any value between −1 and +1. A plot of one value versus the other will show all points consistently stepping upwards or downwards if rho equals +1 or −1. With rho = 0, the points are randomly scattered.
Cronbach's alpha	A measure of the degree of correlation among the answers to a series of questions yielding ordinal responses. Determines whether all the questions are measuring the same thing.
Data transformation	A mathematical manipulation of a data set, generally designed to re-scale it so that it conforms more closely to a normal distribution.
Dependent data	Each value in one data set has a special relationship with a value in another data set. Relatedness usually arises because each participant contributed a value to both data sets. Relatedness can also arise if two values are from separate participants who have been selected as "Matched" based on relevant characteristics. Also called "Related" or "Paired" data.
Descriptive statistics	Values that each summarize some aspect of a dataset, e.g. mean, SD, proportion etc.
Dichotomous	Categorical data that can take only two, mutually exclusive values, e.g. Success/Failure or Live/Dead. Also known as "Binary."

Word	Meaning
Discontinuous	Measurement data that can only take integer (whole number) values. No decimals or fractional values are possible.
Discordant	Term used in relation to McNemar's test. The data for a participant/outcome is discordant if they have different outcomes under the two conditions being studied.
Dot plot	A graph where each dot represents one out of a set of measured values. Useful for describing the distribution of measurement data.
Dunnett's test	A follow up test for one-way ANOVA in which one study group (the Reference group) is compared against all other groups.
Effect size	A measure of how strongly a factor is able to influence the outcome. Important in assessing practical/clinical significance.
Expected frequency	Theoretically calculated frequencies that exactly match the null hypothesis for chi-square tests. These are generated by the computer program as intermediate working. You will not need to calculate them, but problems arise if any of these are less than five.
Exploratory analysis	A statistical analysis carried out in addition to the primary analysis. Must be recognized as multiple testing and likely to raise the risk of false positives. Conclusions should not be relied upon until confirmed by further work. Also known as secondary analysis.
Factor	Something that may be able to influence an outcome. The "cause" part in a cause and effect relationship.
False negative	The factor under investigation does have an influence upon the outcome, but the experimental/trial/survey data does not achieve statistical significance (see *Beta*).
False positive	The factor under investigation has no real influence upon the outcome but the experimental/trial/survey data does indicate statistical significance (see *Alpha*).
Fisher's exact test	Performs the same function as a chi-square test. Useful as an alternative when a chi-square test generates a problem with expected frequencies less than five.
Follow up test	A test performed after a one-way analysis of variance has proved statistically significant. Determines which pairs of study groups show a statistically significantly difference. See *Dunnett's and Tukey's tests*.
Frequency	The number of individuals classified as falling into one category (categorical data) or having one value on an ordinal scale.

Word	Meaning
Friedman's test	A robust, non-parametric equivalent of the repeated measures analysis of variance. Suitable for ordinal data or continuous measured data where the requirement for normal distribution is not met.
G*Power	Software for calculating necessary sample sizes. Freely available from the internet.
Histogram	Similar to a bar chart, but based upon continuous measured data that has been split into a series of ranges. No spaces are left between the bars – this emphasizes the originally continuous nature of the data.
Independent data	No value in one data set has any special relationship with any value in another data set. In a comparative study, each participant belongs to one of the study groups and only contributes a data point to that group's data set. Also known as "Unpaired data."
Independent samples t-test	A statistical test looking for a difference in the mean value of a continuous measured variable in two separate study groups. Assumes normal distributions within both data sets.
Interquartile range	The range between the first and third quartile value. A robust indicator of the variability (dispersion) in a data set.
Kruskal–Wallis test	A robust, non-parametric alternative for one-way analysis of variance. Suitable for ordinal data or continuous measured data that is not normally distributed.
Levels	The number of different possible values for a factor recorded as categorical data. For example, when comparing outcomes for males versus females there are two levels, and when comparing placebo, old drug, and new drug there are three levels.
Likert scale	A scale with between three and seven options ranging from "strongly disagree" to "strongly agree," for participants to indicate the extent to which they agree or disagree with a statement. Generates ordinal data.
Linear relationship	The points on a scatter plot could credibly be fitted by a straight trend line. No clear evidence of a curved (nonlinear) relationship.
Log transform	The logarithms of a series of measured values. When there is a problem with data being positively skewed, the logs often form a distribution much closer to normality. Statistical tests that require normality can then be carried out on the log transformed values rather than using the original values.

Word	Meaning
Logistic regression	A method for determining whether a binary outcome is influenced by (a) one or more continuous measured factors, (b) one or more categorical factors, or (c) a mix of measured and categorical factors. One use is the detection of confounding when several factors apparently influence a categorical outcome.
Long-tailed distribution	A data set that would be normally distributed except for the presence of values, some much lower and some much higher than would be expected based upon the mean and SD of the data set.
Mann–Whitney test	A robust, non-parametric equivalent of the independent samples t-test. Suitable for ordinal data or continuous measured data that is not normally distributed.
Matched pairs	Participants chosen so the first two match each other (in terms of age, sex, etc.), the next two match each other, and so on. Commonly allocated so one member of each pair gets one treatment and the other gets the alternative treatment. Used to obtain related/paired data.
McNemar's test	Test used when there are two study groups with a binary categorical outcome and the outcome data is related/paired (i.e. each participant is studied under both conditions).
Mean	The average of a set of measured values. The sum of all the values divided by the number of observations.
Median	The middle ranking observation. Half of the values will be higher and half lower than the median.
Mode	The most commonly occurring value in a data set.
Monotonic	A relationship between two measured variables. As one variable increases in value, the other either consistently increases or consistently decreases; it does not (for example) increase to a maximum and then decrease.
Multiple testing	Carrying out more than one statistical test. A process that can increase the risk of false positives.
Nominal data	An alternative name for categorical data.
Nonlinear	The points on a scatter plot clearly do not follow a straight trend line. There is a curved relationship.
Non-normal	A data set that would produce a histogram or normal probability plot that is not compatible with a normal distribution.

Word	Meaning
Nonparametric	A test within which no statistical parameters such as the mean or SD are calculated. Data are converted to rank values and all further calculations are based on these. Also known as "distribution free tests." These tests are robust and do not require normal distributions within the data.
Normal distribution	A symmetrical, unimodal distribution of measured values. A histogram of normally distributed data should follow a mathematically defined shape.
Normal probability plot	A plot of the values that would be predicted to be present in a data set (based upon its mean an SD) versus the values actually observed. A line of ideal fit is usually superimposed. Any major deviation of the points from the line indicates non-normality.
Number needed to treat (NNT)	The number of individuals who would have to be transferred from one treatment regime to another in order to produce one additional beneficial outcome (or equivalently, one less detrimental outcome). Calculated as one divided by the ARD, rounded up to the next whole number.
Odds	The likelihood that an event will arise divided by the likelihood that it will not.
Odds ratio (OR)	The odds of an outcome in the experimental or exposed group divided by the odds in the control or unexposed group.
Omnibus test	A test that considers more than two study groups simultaneously. Contrasts with the opposite strategy of sequential testing for differences within each possible pair of groups. Avoids multiple testing.
One-sided	A test for an effect in one (pre-determined) direction. e.g. "Is the mean for group A greater than the mean for group B?" The result can only be significant if there is a difference in the direction indicated (in the above case, the mean for A must be *greater* than the mean for B).
One-tailed	Another term for one-sided.
One-way analysis of variance	A statistical test applied when investigating the effect of a categorical factor with more than two levels upon a continuously varying measured outcome.
Ordinal data	Categorical data with a clear order to the categories. While each step up the scale may be recorded numerically as an increase in the value of one point, It is not necessarily the case that each step is of equal relevance. Examples include age category (Young/Middle aged/Older) and Likert scale responses.

Word	Meaning
Outcome	Data that may be under the influence of something else (the "Factor"). The "effect" part in a cause and effect relationship.
Outlier	One (or a small number of) values that are very high or very low and clearly separate from the main cluster of results.
Paired data	Each value in one data set has a special relationship with a value in another data set. Relatedness usually arises because each participant contributed a value to both data sets. Relatedness can also arise if two values are from separate participants who have been selected as "Matched" based on relevant characteristics. Also called "Dependent" or "Related" data.
Paired t-test	A statistical test looking for differences in a continuous measured outcome when participants are studied under two different conditions (a paired study). Assumes the differences between individuals' measurements in the two conditions/time-points are normally distributed.
Parametric	A test within which statistical parameters such as the mean or SD are calculated. e.g. t-tests and ANOVAs. Generally requires the data to follow a normal distribution.
Pearson correlation	A method to determine how strongly one measured value is related to another. See *Correlation coefficient (r)*.
Point estimate	A sample based estimate of a proportion, mean, or median value for the population. Known to be subject to random sampling error, but the best available estimate of the true value.
Polymodal	Data that falls into two (or more) distinct clusters of higher or lower values, with few (or no) cases with values between the clusters. See also *Bimodal*.
Power	When investigating a factor that does have a real effect on your outcome, power is the likelihood that your sample(s) will achieve statistical significance.
Primary analysis	A single statistical test that will be used to answer your primary research question.
P-value	A measure of how compatible your observed data is with the null hypothesis. Low values indicate that your observed data would be unlikely to arise if the null hypothesis were true, leading to greater credence for the alternative hypothesis.
Quartile	One of a set of three values that will divide ranked, measured data into four equal sized groups. Q1 is the value 25% of the way up the list of ranked values. Q2 (the median) is the middle ranked value and Q3 is 75% of the way up the scale.

Word	Meaning
Rank values	Measured data are sorted from lowest to highest and the first (lowest) value is given rank value 1, then the second is allotted a rank value of 2, and so on. Non-parametric methods always convert results to rank values, and then all further testing uses the rank values.
Reducing a contingency table	Removing the data in one or more rows or columns of a contingency table. See also *Collapsing a contingency table*.
Regression equation	An equation that predicts the value of a continuously varying outcome from that for a continuously varying factor. Can be useful as a measure of effect size: By how much does the outcome vary if the value of the factor increases by one unit?
Related data	Each value in one data set has a special relationship with a value in another data set. Relatedness usually arises because each participant contributed a value to both data sets. Relatedness can also arise if two values are from separate participants who have been selected as "Matched" based on relevant characteristics. Also known as "Dependent" or "Paired" data.
Repeated measures analysis of variance	A statistical test most commonly applied when a continuously varying measured outcome is determined in the same group of subjects at three (or more) time points.
Risk	In statistics, the term "Risk" describes the likelihood of a particular outcome. That outcome is not necessarily harmful or undesirable.
Risk ratio (RR)	The risk of a particular outcome in the experimental or exposed group divided by that for the control or unexposed group.
Robust	A statistical method that will not be greatly affected by non-ideal data sets, e.g., those containing occasional outlying high or low values or that deviate moderately from a normal distribution.
Scale data	The same as continuous measured data (term used in SPSS).
Scatter plot	A graph of one measured variable against that for another. Each point represents the two measured values for one individual.
Scoring	The process of attributing a numerical value to a variable to enable statistical analysis to be performed (particularly needed for ordinal data).

Word	Meaning
Secondary analyses	Statistical analyses that are additional to the primary analysis. These will increase the risk of false positives, so the results of secondary analyses need to be treated with caution and may need to be confirmed by further work. Also known as "Exploratory analyses."
Significance (Practical or Clinical)	A determination of whether the effect of a factor upon the outcome is large enough to be of practical significance: Does it justify recommending a change to professional practice or public policy?
Significance (Statistical)	A determination of whether the data provides evidence against the null hypothesis and thereby markedly increases the credibility of the alternative hypothesis. It only signifies increased confidence that there is an effect; it says nothing about the size and practical significance of the effect.
Significant digits	Number of non-zero digits reported. See Section 6.4 for a full description.
Skewed distribution	A distribution of measured data where most of the observations are at the low end of the range of observed values with small numbers of much higher values (positive skew) or the opposite pattern – mainly high values, but a few much lower ones (negative skew).
Spearman correlation	A robust, non-parametric equivalent of Pearson correlation. Especially useful where one (or both) sets of measured data are ordinal. See *Correlation coefficient (rho)*.
SPSS	A computer program marketed by IBM, the original name for which is Statistical Package for the Social Sciences, used across a wide range of disciplines for data storage and statistical analysis.
Stacked bar chart	Used for categorical or ordinal data. The various categories are each represented by a bar, and these are then stacked on top of each other rather than side-by-side. Can be used to represent either the counts or proportions in each category. If proportions are represented, the sample size must be indicated.
Standard deviation (SD)	An indicator of the degree of variability of individual values around the overall mean within a set of measured data.
Statistical power	The likelihood that a given experimental design (including some pre-determined sample size) will result in a conclusion of statistical significance. The definition assumes that, within the population being studied, the factor under investigation really does have an effect upon the relevant outcome.

Word	Meaning
t-Test	See *Independent samples t-test* and *Paired t-test*.
Tukey' test	A follow up test for one-way analysis of variance in which all possible pairs of study groups are compared.
Two-sided	A test for an effect of a factor upon the outcome that does not specify the direction of change. For example "Is the mean value for a measured outcome different for a new treatment regime and an older one?" The result will be significant if the mean is either markedly lower or higher with the new regime.
Two-tailed	Same as two-sided.
Unimodal	A distribution of measured data where values vary but they all cluster around a single point. The data does not split into distinct clusters of high and low values.
Unpaired	No value in one data set has any special relationship with any value in another data set. In a comparative study, each participant belongs to one of the study groups and only contributes a data point to that group's data set. Also known as "Independent data."
Validation	A process whereby a research instrument is subjected to rigorous tests to determine its usefulness for measuring or assessing a behavioral, attitudinal, or clinical feature of respondents.
Visual analog scale (VAS)	A measurement instrument for subjective outcomes. Participants report their level of the variable (e.g. pain or agreement with a statement) by indicating a position along a line between two end-points. The distance of their mark along the line provides the outcome measure.
Welch's test	A modified version of the independent samples t-test or one-way analysis of variance that does not require equal standard deviations in the study groups being compared.
Wilcoxon rank sum test	An alternative name for the Mann–Whitney test. The term is best avoided as it is too similar to "Wilcoxon signed rank test."

Videos

Number	Title	Description
1.1	SPSS_Basics	The absolute basics of using SPSS
2.1	Normality_ Testing	Using SPSS to determine whether measured data follows a normal distribution, and log transformation to improve normality
3.1	Descriptives Proportions	Using SPSS to obtain the mean, 95% confidence interval for the mean, standard deviation, quartiles, and means and proportion for categorised data
7.1	ChiSquare_ SampSize	Using G*Power for chi-square sample size calculation
7.2	ChiSquare Test	Using SPSS for contingency tables, chi-square test, Yates correction, Fisher's exact test and Relative Risk etc. plus confidence intervals
7.3	Detecting Confounding	Using SPSS for logistic regression to detect confounding
8.1	t-test_SampSize	Using G*Power to calculate necessary sample size for a t-test
8.2	t-test	Using SPSS to perform the t-test and (if necessary) switch to Welch's test
9.1	Mann Whitney Test	Using SPSS for the Mann–Whitney Test
10.1	ANOVA	Using SPSS to perform a one-way analysis of variance and follow up tests
11.1	Kruskal–Wallis	Using SPSS to carry out a Kruskal–Wallis test

A Practical Approach to Using Statistics in Health Research: From Planning to Reporting, First Edition. Adam Mackridge and Philip Rowe.
© 2018 John Wiley & Sons, Inc. Published 2018 by John Wiley & Sons, Inc.
Companion website: www.wiley.com/go/Mackridge/
APracticalApproachtoUsingStatisticsinHealthResearch

Number	Title	Description
12.1	McNemar	Using a spreadsheet to calculate necessary sample size for a McNemar test, and how to perform the test using SPSS
13.1	Paired_t_SampSize	Using G*Power for paired-t sample size calculation
13.2	Paired_t	Using SPSS to perform a paired t-test
14.1	Wilcoxon_Signed_Rank	Using SPSS to carry out a Wilcoxon signed rank test
14.1	Wilcoxon Signed Rank	Using SPSS to carry out a Wilcoxon signed rank test
15.1	RepMeasures	Using SPSS to perform a repeated measures analysis of variance and Bonferroni corrected follow up tests
16.1	Friedman	Using SPSS to perform Friedman's test and follow up tests
17.1	Pearson Correlation Regression	Using SPSS to carry out Pearson correlation and regression analyses
17.2	Pearson_SampSize	Calculating the sample size required for a Pearson Correlation using G*Power
18.1	Spearman Correlation	Using SPSS to carry out Spearman correlation
19.1	Logistic Regression	Using SPSS for binary logistic regression
20.1	Cronbach	Using SPSS to calculate Cronbach's Alpha, including sequential removal of each item

Index